HEALTHY [illegible]YLE

AFTER 40

~An Unconventional Guide To Healthy Lifestyle After 40 Without Feeling on a Diet~

By,

Tamaya Eden

This report is towards furnishing precise and solid data concerning the point and issue secured. The production is sold with the possibility that the distributor isn't required to render bookkeeping, formally allowed, or something else, qualified administrations. On the off chance that exhortation is important, lawful, or proficient, a rehearsed individual in the calling ought to be requested.

The Declaration of Principles, which was also recognized and endorsed by the Committee of the American Bar Association and the Committee of Publishers and Associations.

The data gave in this is expressed, to be honest, and predictable, in that any risk, as far as absentmindedness or something else, by any utilization or maltreatment of any approaches, procedures, or bearings contained inside is the singular and articulate obligation

CONTENTS

~INTRODUCTION~

Good health is a condition of full physical, emotional, and social wellbeing, not just the absence of disease or illness. This entails maintaining a well-balanced diet, exercising regularly, abstaining from cigarettes and other substances, and having plenty of rest.

To remain in good working order, our bodies need a combination of protein, carbohydrates, fat, vitamins, minerals, and water.

If you don't strike the right balance, your wellbeing will suffer.

A healthy diet entails only consuming as many calories as you burn during the day.

If you consume more calories than you spend, any excess will be stored as fat.

Have you ever found that your perception of a healthy lifestyle varies from someone else's? It could mean so many things to different people, which is a good thing. It's also a bit perplexing. Eating nutritious foods and becoming aerobically active as a way of life are the most clear descriptions of a healthy lifestyle.

However, two people rarely make the same food decisions or participate in the same activities. Ginny, for example, eats raw foods and goes for a run nearly every day of the week. Margaret likes pasta and grilled foods, and she has learned that eating whole wheat pasta and lean meats is a safe way of doing so. Kayaking, cycling, Tai Chi, and gardening are among her favorite pastimes. Robert loves swimming, dancing, and hiking, and he consumes a lot of complex carbohydrates. They're all living good lives, but they're not the same.

So, how do you know if you are eating and doing things that are good for you?

There are many methods for determining this.

One place to begin is to educate yourself on the fundamentals of good nutrition and aerobic exercise. The food pyramid is a good point to began learning about nutrition because it is focused on consuming a variety of foods in moderation and adhering to healthy guidelines rather than on following a strict diet. Knowing the goal heart rate zones is a good way to learn about aerobic fitness. Heart rate charts can be found on the walls of gyms and on the Internet, and they teach you how to gauge and assess the ideal exercise intensity. The food pyramid and heart rate zones are tools that can help you make your own choices about which foods to consume and how much exercise to do.

The following step is to pay attention to how your body feels. Feed if you're hungry. Stop if you're full. If you're tired, see what happens if you rest versus if you do a little more. If you're in pain and don't know what to do, seek assistance. Start moving if you're out of shape. You'll get hints on what's right for you if you pay attention to your own body. Our natural instinct is to ignore the signs, but you'll soon discover that this isn't a wise decision. Your physical symptoms will worsen before you actually pay attention and start making healthy lifestyle changes, as I have experienced firsthand.

The third choice is to seek advice from a specialist you can trust and who will listen when you say something does not feel right. Be mindful that not all practitioners are trustworthy or can act in your best interests. If your instinct tells you not to do a particular thing, listen to it. Following the instructions of a personal trainer, I injured my back, and some of my clients have done the same.

Living a balanced lifestyle means being less physically and emotionally stressed. Having a good night's sleep, drinking plenty of water, limiting alcohol consumption to moderate levels, and taking a multivitamin can all help reduce stress. Another important aspect is how you react to circumstances. You can be frustrated and nervous when stuck in traffic or relaxed and focused on something more fun. Even if it doesn't look that way, it is a decision.

PART I

~BRAIN CHANGE BEFORE BODY CHANGE~

Anything you do involve the brain.

All you do, feel and think is controlled by your brain. You should thank the brain for what you see when you look in the mirror. If your belly bulges over your belt buckle or your waistline is slim and toned is essentially decided by your brain. If your skin appears new and dewy or wrinkled is largely determined by your brain.

Your brain determines whether you feel energized or groggy when you wake up. When it comes to choosing between leftover pizza and low-fat yogurt and fruit for breakfast, it is your brain that makes the decision. If you go to the gym or sit at the screen to update your Facebook profile is determined by your brain. It's also your brain that makes you want to smoke a cigarette or drink a few cups of coffee.

TAKE ACTION

Remember that your brain is involved in every decision you make, every bite of food you take, every cigarette you smoke, every worrying thought you have, every workout you skip, and every alcoholic beverage you drink.

Your way of thinking, feeling, eating, exerting and even making love depends on how your brain works at any moment. The brain has a much deeper effect on the body. It is important to your health and wellbeing overall. Your brain is at the core of it all, whether you live a long and prosperous life, suffer from a chronic illness, or have your days cut short by a horrific disease. In reality, researchers from the University of Cambridge in England discovered that bad decisions made with one's brain cut one's life span by fourteen years. At the age of sixty, people who drank heavily, smoked, didn't exercise and ate poorly had the same chance of dying as people who lived a balanced lifestyle until they were seventy-four. Your brain's actions can either take away or add years to your life!

Your body looks and feels healthier when your brain is working properly. When your brain is messed up, it affects how you look and feel.

It's much easier to have the best body when you have a balanced brain. You are more likely to adhere to a diet, workout schedule and develop healthy lifestyle habits as your brain is functioning at its best. This translates to a slimmer, trimmer body, a more youthful look, lighter skin, increased immunity, fewer headaches, lower back pain, and better overall health.

A disturbed brain, on the other hand, often leads to physical issues. Extra pounds, wrinkles, chronic pain, and other health problems can all be related to how the brain works. When your brain isn't functioning properly, you're more likely to make bad eating decisions, skip the gym, and engage in unhealthy habits.

Jim, a divorced engineer in his fifties, stands five foot ten inches tall and weighs about 260 pounds. He tries to diet, but he can't seem to keep it up. Jim gets up every morning intending to eat healthily for the day, but he never gets around to preparing his meals or filling the refrigerator. He's hungry as lunchtime comes, so he stops at the first fast-food joint he sees and buys a cheeseburger and fries. When he gets home from work, he looks into an empty refrigerator before ordering pizza from a nearby delivery service.

Mary seems to be older than her forty-three years, with three small children, a stressful career, and a troubled marriage. She'd like to reclaim her youthful appearance but hasn't been able to do so with the beauty counter's creams and lotions. She seldom gets more than a few hours of sleep at night, and if she's depressed, tired, crazy, or sad, she turns to a cigarette and a glass of wine—or two, three, four, or even the entire bottle. Smoking and drinking temporarily calms her nerves and helps her feel better.

Sandra, who is twenty-eight years old, wishes she had a stronger body. She needs to tone and tighten the 135 pounds she wears on her five-foot-six-inch frame, even though she isn't technically overweight. She acknowledges that exercise will help her accomplish her objectives, but she can't seem to summon the energy or encouragement to go to the gym. Sarah also suffers from anxiety and nervousness, and she is constantly concerned about what could go wrong with her life.

Jim, Mary and Sandra have attributed their issues to a lack of willpower or laziness for years, but this isn't always the case. Their minds are to blame for their failure to attain the body they crave. Jack's lack of planning and poor follow-through are both symptoms of low activity in the prefrontal cortex, a part of the brain (PFC). This portion of the brain is responsible for goal-setting, forethought, impulse control, and follow-through. It's very difficult to be competitive when this area isn't working properly.

Smoking or drinking to relieve stress, which is preventing Mary from achieving the youthful appearance she desires, can indicate excessive activity in the brain's deep limbic system. This portion of the brain is responsible for deciding your emotional sound. When it is less busy, people have a more upbeat, optimistic attitude. Negativity and feelings of distress or sadness may take over when it is heated or overactive, leading you to seek solace in smoking, alcohol, or narcotics.

CHAPTER 1

~WHAT ARE THE BENEFITS OF A HEALTHY LIFESTYLE?~

What Is a HEALTHY LIFESTYLE?

1. A way of life that decreases the risk of being chronically ill or dying early. While not all illness and disease can be prevented, a significant number of deaths, especially those caused by coronary heart disease and lung cancer, can be avoided. Certain forms of activity have been linked to serious illness and early death in scientific research.

2. A way of life that helps you to enjoy more facets of it. It's not just about preventing disease or sickness when it comes to good health. It also pertains to one's physical, emotional, and social wellbeing.

3. A way of life that benefits the whole family. When you live a healthy lifestyle, you set a better example for those in your family, especially your children. You can also provide them with a better world in which to grow up. You will be contributing to their wellness and enjoyment of life now and in the future by assisting them in adopting a healthy lifestyle.

By definition and realization, wellbeing is a natural part of life. The secret of " jivem shardah shatam " - a hundred years of robust, balanced, peaceful, and creative life - was attributed by the ancient Indians to the complete harmony of the mode of living with Nature and the divine inheritance of life. Staying safe is influenced by one's way of life. We come strictly and regularly to maintain our physical health because that is what we have placed in our bodies. When it comes to our diet, we recognize the importance of eating fresh, whole foods and a commitment to eliminating foods that are high in fat and oil. Yet, more than anything else, physical exercise assists in the prevention of illness and keeps us strong and secure in the future. What does it mean to live a safe life? A healthy workout program requires workouts that are suitable for your current health and lifestyle. If you're currently seated, ease into a workout regimen by incorporating a small amount of exercise into your everyday routine. Raising your strength and conditioning as you develop is a fantastic workout that will benefit your whole body. Beginners can easily overcome fitness and fitness issues. Begin by walking for a few minutes each day, gradually increasing your pace and distance until you feel good.

A lifestyle is described as a person's way of life in sociology. A sedentary lifestyle is one of the huge risk factors for a number of diseases. Psychotic lifestyle is a psychological term for a way of life that includes any or unusual physical activity. A couch potato is an individual who leads a sedentary lifestyle and can be found in both developed and developing countries. Sitting sports, reading, watching television, and using computers for a long time have little to no intense physical activity. Many preventable causes of death can be attributed to a sedentary lifestyle. A seamless lifestyle is one in which a person does not participate in sufficient physical activity, despite the fact that this is commonly considered to be a healthy lifestyle. Sedentary lifestyle people are defined by long periods of sitting, whether in front of a television or a computer screen. Sedentary lifestyle people ignore physical activity and engage in activities that seldom require physical discomfort. According to a new report, leading a sedentary lifestyle is potentially more harmful to one's health than smoking.

Lots of studies have been carried out on the impact of a sedentary lifestyle on individuals all over the world. The following are some highlights of these studies:

The most visible consequence of a sedentary lifestyle is the size of your trouser. Since you are eating a lot of calories but not burning any of them, these calories are stored as fat in your body. And this is just the beginning of the issues. Your heart requires enough blood supply from the blood vessels to function properly (coronary arteries). Leading blood circulation will slow down, stiffen, and block your blood vessels if you live a sedentary lifestyle. It can lead to arteriosclerosis and cardiac arrest in serious cases. According to a study, the risk of death from heart failure in your Middle Ages can be as high as 52 percent for men and 28 percent for women due to a lack of physical activity. Frequent exercise aids in the management of blood glucose levels. According to studies performed by Duke University Medical Center researchers, vigorous exercise will boost the body's ability to regulate blood glucose levels significantly. Blood sugar levels have risen as a result of a lack of exercise, putting more strain on the pancreas (which hides the insides of the hormone insulin). Type 2 diabetes is more likely as a result of this.

Reduced activity raises the risk of contracting such cancers, such as breast cancer, colon cancer, and other deadly tumors. Physical inactivity can be as high as 45 percent for men and 28 percent for women, according to a study conducted by Hong Kong University.

Inactivity for a long period of time weakens your bones because they are no longer challenged to sustain the structure of your body. Inactive lifestyles can cause arthritis and osteoporosis, which cause bones to become brittle and weak. Your muscles are like a car battery; they need to be charged on a regular basis to keep the car running. You have less muscle capacity, which has the potential if you live a more sedentary lifestyle. You have less muscular muscles and the ability to function on a daily basis. Being a couch potato has a major impact on the wellbeing of your posture and spinal cord. Sitting all day will weaken and stiffen your hip flexors and hamstrings while also weakening and stiffening the back muscles that protect your spinal cord.

A sedentary lifestyle places no physical strain on the body. As a consequence, the body does not feel like relaxing, which often leads to sleeping issues and, in extreme cases, insomnia. Researchers in Norway discovered that those who did not exercise regularly had a 14 percent higher chance of experiencing a non-migraine headache.

Of course, if you've been living a sedentary lifestyle for a long time, getting back into shape can be a challenge. However, if you progressively incorporate high-intensity activities into your daily routine, such as biking, ironing, dog walking, walking, riding, and so on, you will be well on your way to living a proactive and safe lifestyle. It may be from.

Living a healthy lifestyle

We all know that staying healthy requires a lot of exercise and adhering to a strict diet plan. However, many of us enjoy this grandmother's advice: we listen to it but forget it and return to our old habits. We enjoy our sedentary lifestyle because it does not require us to do many things; we spend far too much time in front of the television, and if that isn't enough, we supplement it with a diet rich in fast food.

What Are the Benefits of a Healthy Lifestyle?

The good of a healthy lifestyle are becoming more pronounced as our perception of our bodies has changed over time, as well as for reasons we can immerse the body at least once yearly to eliminate harmful bacteria. Insects, too, can be found in our intestines.

A balanced lifestyle has many advantages for people of all ages, weights, and skills. But for now, consider these eight straightforward advantages of leading a balanced lifestyle. Good health is not something you can purchase in a drugstore or department store, but it can be accomplished by following a collective pattern of health-related actions based on the choices made from the available options. Following this point, if you want to reap the benefits of a balanced lifestyle, incorporate some healthy habits into your regular or weekly routines, such as eating well and exercising. Other advantages include lower health-care rates, fewer accidents and injuries, fewer shospitals, remaining working, and improved employee-employer ties.

Weight management is essential for maintaining all of the health benefits of a healthier lifestyle; even a ten percent weight loss reduces the risk of heart disease and other obesity-related diseases. Obesity / excess weight is the second leading cause of many childhood illnesses, including osteoporosis, sleep apnea, type 2 diabetes, asthma, high blood pressure and cholesterol, skin disorders, and emotional and psychological issues. Weight lifting, such as walking and strength training, can help to initiate and/or avoid osteoporosis, and some evidence indicates that by doing so, bone mass can eventually become bone, and the disease can begin to reverse.

Weight loss, stress reduction, enhanced wellbeing, increased self-image and self-esteem, and better physical work are some other advantages. While medicines can sometimes bring cholesterol levels back to normal, diet and exercise benefits are not included in medicines. They lower blood pressure, help people lose weight and lower the risk of diabetes. I'm a high-risk candidate for a sedentary lifestyle disorder. Exercise and a balanced diet help the body use insulin more effectively, which can aid in the regulation, reduction, and prevention of a variety of diseases. Reduce the risk of heart disease by learning to exercise, quit smoking, eat more fiber and low-fat foods, maintain a healthy weight, and cope with stress. For different aesthetic, social, and medical purposes, we all want a trim and balanced body.

A practice program was shown to substantially reduce LDL cholesterol and other dangerous factors in patients with cardiovascular disease in a study performed by Tufts University at the New England Medical Center among patients with cardiovascular disease. More than what counseling can offer. Even minimal weight loss can lower medical and pharmacy costs, minimize the need for bariatric surgery, and cure co-ailments such as asthma, high blood pressure, and diabetes.

Wellness is about feeling at peace with your own skin: your body, your mind, and your surroundings. A person's lifespan can be increased by leading a healthy lifestyle. And, while catching infectious diseases such as colds or fluids is often unavoidable, it is comforting to know that it is a safer way of recovering, you should ask yourself why you're as beneficial as possible to live every day. It is not to be taken. Many people today have the problem of being so preoccupied with working and/or caring for others that they forget their own health and wellbeing. Make sure the heart and bones are in good shape and maintain them to reap the benefits of a balanced lifestyle. Taking good care of yourself is the sole way to ensuring good health. The stakes are high, but the possible rewards include preventing premature death, unnecessary disease and disability, lowering health-care costs, and ensuring a high quality of life in old age. You are doing who you are when you live a balanced lifestyle, and you don't have to be self-conscious about things you wouldn't do if you did not think about your lifestyle.

With a healthier lifestyle and more power over your life, you can work with your body to reclaim those facets of your life that you can. You can monitor your sleep habits and feel good all day long if you live a balanced lifestyle. All works together to understand and support other aspects of your lifestyle while you live a balanced lifestyle.

Healthy weight loss, healthy eating, and exercise habits have been scientifically proven to boost health and help manage common chronic diseases including high cholesterol, hypertension, diabetes, stress, and general stamina deficiency.

A balanced lifestyle also provides a steady supply of endurance and strength, allowing you to engage in activities and improve your versatility. A healthy lifestyle includes a well-balanced and varied diet that provides the body with vital nutrients and energy. You have the potential to be trained to help you develop muscles that protect your bones and joints, decreasing the risk of falling and fracture. Cardiovascular exercise, also known as aerobic exercise, improves the heart muscles, increasing the heart's effectiveness. As we get older, our bones lose a lot of bio-biological power. Weight lifting, walking and strength training, can help to initiate and/or avoid osteoporosis, and some evidence indicates that by doing so, bone mass can eventually become bone, and the disease can begin to reverse. The good news is that you wouldn't have to train like an Olympic athlete to reap the rewards of leading a balanced lifestyle.

As part of your regular or weekly routines, mystery and rationality are repeating a preferred safe pattern. It is a way of life to live a safe lifestyle.

A safe lifestyle is one that reduces the chances of being chronically ill or dying prematurely. While not all diseases are preventable, many deaths, particularly those caused by coronary heart disease and lung cancer, can be prevented. Certain forms of behavior have been described in scientific studies as contributing to the development of noncommunicable diseases and early death.

It's not just about preventing illness when it comes to good health. Physical, emotional, and social wellbeing are all factors. When a healthier lifestyle is adopted, it provides a more positive role model for other family members, especially children. This book aims at assisting readers in changing their habits and improving their health in order to live healthier and longer lives.

CHAPTER 2

~40 YEARS, A MOMENT OF BALANCE?~

It's a plain fact that most women despise the prospect of growing older. I know, it's a shocker. It's easy to understand why, considering society's general attitude toward aging. Nonetheless, there are some truly remarkable aspects of completing your fifth, sixth, seventh, and beyond decades. One of the most significant? No twenty-something may demand knowledge based on life experience.

By the time you're 40, you've amassed a wealth of insights about everything from how to get over a lost love to what really constitutes happiness. From a combination of lifestyle gurus and, of course, women over 40 themselves, we've compiled the top pieces of information experts believe women over 40 possess.

Perfection Isn't Necessary!

Cara Maksimow, LCSW, CPC, a therapist, Coach, speaker, and author: "When we are young, so many ladies strive to be perfect and set unrealistic expectations on themselves."
"This can lead to black-and-white thinking and anger."

"It can trigger undue stress and low self-esteem if I'm not okay, I'm failing. When we get older, the more we realize it can be beautiful to lack a perfection."

The Influence of Self-Talk

"I have spent so much of my twenties and thirties being hurt and offended by other people or concerned about what others think about me," says Limor Weinstein, psychotherapist, eating disorder counseling and founder of the LW Wellness Network. "Back then, I wish I had known what I know now. When I was 42, I was so much nicer than I was, and I was much happier! I now understand that my own emotions are solely responsible for me and that I can transform my negative thinking into positive ones which help me develop – and help others to grow in turn."

Winning Isn't the Only Thing That Matters

The author and producer of the Superior Self series, KJ Landis, says, "To be a participant and to be surrounded by similar people is a reward in yourself" when you are in the 40s. "In my 40s, I ran 16 marathons (beginning with 40) and was ecstatic about the spirit of the crowd, not to mention the fact that I finished each!"

Aging is an inevitable part of life

And the alternative is much more dangerous! "I'm not saying I want to age gracefully (I spend enough money on serums and creams each month), but I am proud of the life experiences, both positive and challenging, that those lines represent," says Monique Honaman, author of The High Road Has Less Traffic: Truthful Advice on the Journey Through Love and Divorce. What is her recommendation? "Take control of your lines and the story they tell."

When to Accept No as an Answer

It's not always worth it to fight. "We've learned to embrace the answer and move on after 40 years of hearing no or being told no," says Tracee Dunblazier, a spiritual empath and relationship coach. "We have no power over anything but ourselves.

Reasons Why You Shouldn't Take No for an Answer

Women over 40, on the other hand, know that something is really worth fighting for. "By the age of 40, most women have seen gender disparity in some way or another—whether we've stood up for ourselves or cheered on the brave women we know who have," Dunblazier says.

Style Is a Personal Preference

Now is the time to put on whatever you want. "Women in their 40s can express themselves by wearing what feels authentic to them, regardless of social trends, views, or 'likes' of others," says Dr.

Karin Luise, author of The Fatherless Daughter Project. Women over 40 are well aware that the 30 Ugliest Dresses Ever are not to be worn.

Minor Issues That Should Remain Minor

"'Don't sweat the small stuff,' as the saying goes. It is right "CEO, licensed counselor, and executive leadership consultant Allison Kanter Agliata agrees. "When you get to the age of forty, you realize that not every war is worth fighting. Some people aren't worth your time and resources, and others aren't a priority."

Don't take anything you hear as gospel

"Personality is like a software program, furnished with prime values and boundaries, which plays over and over," according to Aimee Bernstein, a psychotherapist, executive coach and author of Stress Less Achieve More: Easy ways of turning pressure into a productive force in your life. "We will live a small life and spend time proving that we are right, as long as we hold fast to our beliefs." Forties, women know how to let down and move on with negative feelings.

It's the little things that make life worthwhile

Life consists of tiny moments like these. "It's not just the small things that make a difference; it's doing them on a regular basis," says Mary Black, a lifestyle coach. "Eating well, exercising, hugging people we care for, sharing a smile, and being kind to others (and ourselves) has a much greater effect on our lives and the lives of others than we knew."

It's All Right to Take Your Time

"Younger women may be frantically pursuing what they or others want for them career advancement, a partner and family, and so on. Until taking their next move, women in their 40s have time to slow down and reassess what is important to them. "Dr. Rosenfeld elucidates the situation. "Things aren't as hurried or time-sensitive, so they have more time to investigate and reflect on what feels authentically good for them."

The Importance of a Good Night's Sleep

"Truly, nothing positive happens after midnight," Cheryl Cieko, an architect specializing in health and wellness, says of her post-40 attitude toward sleep. "Sleep is both safe and enjoyable. More of it is needed."

It Is Important To Be Well-Informed About Your Health

"There isn't time to waste in getting the preventative medical care you need and deserve once you're in your 40s," says Kanesha Baynard, a lifestyle and innovation coach.

It's impossible to please everybody

Life is far too brief. "If I could alter the hands of time, I'd spend the endless hours I spent trying to impress other people on the people in my life that I truly enjoy being around," Weinstein says.

Flossing Is Really Important

Along with all of the other good practices that experts have long recommended. "It wasn't until I turned 40 and noticed that my gums were receding that I realized how necessary flossing is," Honaman says. You have the self-discipline once you hit 40 to adopt healthy behaviors that might have seemed inconvenient a decade ago.

You're solely responsible for your own choices

Gone are the days when you'd do something just because someone else told you to. "Women over 40 will not do what others tell them is 'healthy,' but rather what makes them feel good," Dr. Luise says.

When to Hold them and When to Fold them

Women over 40 are very good at understanding when to hang on to feelings and when to let them go. They understand that resentment and grudges aren't constructive or useful. They've seen and seen enough to know what really matters.

There's Nothing Wrong With Spending the Night At Home

Women in their forties learn that, while socializing with friends is enjoyable and satisfying, partying late brings more harm than good. Ypu could invite friends over for a peaceful night in or spend their nights engaging in self-care activities (reading, relaxing, taking a bath). In any case, they'll get more sleep, won't be hungover, and will be energized and refreshed the next day.

It's Not Enough for Special Occasions to Feel Good

Pleasure should not be reserved for weekends, special holidays, or vacations. Pleasure should be a part of your everyday routine. You know in your forties that you have total control of how you want to feel.

Downtime Has Its Advantages

We always find ourselves rushing from one task to the next because modern life puts such pressure on us to do, create, and succeed.

We can easily lose our sense of self in the process. Downtime allows us to reconnect with our true self.

We are open and comfortable when we are not doing something, and as a result, perspectives and innovative ideas find their way to us.

Life Isn't a Destination; It's a Journey

As the journey progresses, the grey hairs begin to accumulate, the kids pass out, and the mates develop. Enjoy the present moment, as well as any other moment along the way. Nobody can tell you where the finish line is.

It's Necessary to Be Versatile

"When I was younger, I was so stubborn in my daily life," Landis says. "I wanted to get my way, or I'd be miserable. I'm currently learning how to get 'flexi-legs.' Why should I be worried about matters about which I have no control?"

It's Important to Have Your Own Life

Many women sacrifice so much for their significant others, their children, their jobs, and their volunteer work that by the time they reach 40, they haven't done anything for themselves in years. Retirement and empty-nesting are closer than you would expect. That you do not wake up one day, look around, and wonder who that guy in the mirror is, find out who you are and what you enjoy.

Your Health Is More Important Now Than It Has Ever Been

"Menopause is just around the corner," Honaman says, "which means muscle mass and bone density both begin to decrease." This is something that most women in their 40s are conscious of.

"That was a much more effective motivator for me to go to the gym and pursue a healthier lifestyle than turning up at the beach in a bikini had been decades before. It's not all about vanity; the stakes for one's wellbeing are higher than they've ever been."

Look for the Positive in Negative Circumstances

Things are bound to go wrong, but women over the age of 40 know how to handle them. Bernstein observes, "If you can find the main learning in a tough situation, you can emerge stronger, more evolved."

"If you've got the eyes to see and the ears to hear, any difficult circumstance and person can be your teacher. It is easier to move forward and learn faster if you go with the rhythm of the situation rather than battling it."

There's Still Time to Change

Most people believe that by the time they hit their 40s, their personalities are set in stone, but research indicates that this is not the case.

According to scientists, people will become more cooperative, agreeable, and responsible well into their 40s and beyond, which is likely why women over 40 are continually evolving.

Self-Love Is the Key to a Lot of Your Problems

Particularly ones that have to do with relationships. No one else will love you unless you first love yourself. If being alone is boring, it's likely that you are boring as well. Take care of your amusement.

IT'S ILLOGICAL TO PRETEND TO BE ANYONE OTHER THAN YOURSELF

At 40, you know you only get one shot at life, and you'd better make the most of it. We take out time to focus on ourselves and find out what we really want in life.

A priority is living an authentic life and making a difference in the world.

CHAPTER 3

~ASPECTS OF HEALTH~

What is the concept of good health?

A condition of full mental and physical wellbeing is referred to as wellness. Healthcare exists to assist individuals in maintaining their full health.

Healthcare expenditures in the US were $3.5 trillion in 2017, according to the Centers for Disease Control and Prevention (CDC).

Despite this spending, Americans have a shorter life span than people in other developed countries. This is as a result of a number of factors, including healthcare access and lifestyle decisions.

Stress management and enjoying a longer, more active life are both dependent on good health. We will discuss the sense of good health, the different types of health that an individual should recognize, and how to maintain good health in this ebook.

What exactly is health?

The World Health Organization (WHO) described health in 1948 with a term that is still used today.
"Health isn't just the lack of illness or infirmity; it is a condition of full physical, emotional, and social wellbeing."

The WHO clarified the situation in 1986, saying, *"A resource for daily life, not the aim of living." Health is a positive philosophy that emphasizes social and personal capital in addition to physical abilities."*
This implies that wellbeing is a means to an end, rather than an end in itself, for an individual's role in society. A healthy lifestyle avails you the opportunity to live a complete, fulfilling life.
Researchers writing in The Lancet in 2009 described health as the body's ability to adjust to new threats and illnesses.
They base this concept on the fact that modern science has made substantial progress in disease knowledge over the last few decades by learning how diseases function, finding new ways to delay or avoid them, and recognizing that a pathology-free environment might not be feasible.

Types

The two aspects of wellbeing that are most often debated are mental and physical health.

Overall wellbeing is influenced by spiritual, mental, and financial wellbeing. These have been related by medical professionals to reduced stress and enhanced mental and physical health.

People in better financial health, for instance, may be less worried about money and have the ability to purchase fresh food on a more regular basis. Those who have good spiritual health can experience a sense of peace and intent, which can help them maintain good mental health.

Inequities in health have different effects on each of us. Visit our dedicated hub to learn more about health inequalities and what we can do to address them.

Physical health

The bodily functions and processes of an individual in good physical health are likely to be at their best.

This is due to more than just a lack of illness. Regular exercise, a well-balanced diet, and proper rest are all beneficial to one's health. When medical care is required to preserve the equilibrium, people obtain it.

To reduce the risk of illness, physical wellbeing entails leading a healthy lifestyle. Physical exercise, for example, can protect and enhance a person's breathing and heart rate endurance, as well as muscle strength, flexibility, and body composition.

Taking care of one's physical health and wellbeing also entails lowering the likelihood of injury or illness, such as:

- ✓ reducing occupational risks;
- ✓ using contraceptives while having intercourse;
- ✓ maintaining effective hygiene;
- ✓ avoiding cigarettes, alcohol, or illicit drugs;
- ✓ getting the recommended vaccinations for a particular disease or country while traveling.

Physical and mental health can work together to increase a person's overall quality of life.

According to a 2008 report, mental illness, such as depression, can increase the risk of substance use disorders. This could have a negative impact on one's physical health.

Mental health

Mental wellbeing refers to a person's emotional, social, and psychological well-being, according to the United States Department of Health and Human Services. As part of a full, active lifestyle, mental wellbeing is just as critical as physical health.

Since many psychiatric diagnoses are based on an individual's understanding of their experience, defining mental health is more difficult than defining physical health.

However, due to advances in science, physicians can now detect certain physical signs of mental illness in CT scans and genetic tests.

The lack of depression, anxiety, or another condition is not the only criterion for good mental health. It also depends on a person's willingness to:

- ✓ appreciate life;
- ✓ recover from adversity;
- ✓ adjust to adversity;
- ✓ feel comfortable and confident;
- ✓ reach their full potential;
- ✓ balance various aspects of life, such as family and finances.

Physical and mental health are inextricably related. For example, if a chronic condition makes it difficult for a person to perform daily activities, it may lead to depression and stress. These feelings may be a result of financial struggles or a loss of mobility.

Depression or anorexia, for example, may have an effect on body weight and general function.

It's critical to see "health" as a whole rather than as a set of disparate factors. All aspects of health are interconnected, and people should strive for overall wellbeing and balance as the foundations of good health.

Factors that contribute to good health

(A variety of factors influence one's health)

- ***Genetic factors***

An individual is born with a number of different genes. An odd genetic pattern or change in some people may result in less-than-optimal health. People will inherit genes from their parents that put them at higher risk for certain diseases.

- ***Environmental factors***

Environmental conditions have an effect on one's health. It is sometimes enough for the climate to have an impact on one's wellbeing. In certain cases, an environmental stimulus may cause illness in someone who has a genetic predisposition to a disease.

Access to healthcare is important, but according to the ***WHO***, the following factors may have a greater effect on health:

• A person's residence; the state of the environment; genetics; their income; their level of education; and their employment status.

<u>These could be grouped into the following categories:</u>

• Social and economic conditions: This may include a family's or community's financial situation, as well as the social culture and quality of relationships.

• The physical environment: This covers things like how many germs are present in a given location and how much waste is present.

• Attributes and habits of a person: The genetic makeup of a person as well as their lifestyle decisions may have an effect on their overall health.

According to some research, people with a higher socioeconomic status (SES) are more likely to have good health, a good education, a well-paid career, and be able to afford good healthcare in times of sickness or injury.

They also say that people with low socioeconomic status are more likely to experience stress as a result of everyday life stressors, including financial difficulties, marital problems, and unemployment.

Marginality and inequality, for example, may have an effect on the risk of poor health for people with lower SES. A low socioeconomic status also means restricted access to healthcare. People in developing countries with universal healthcare have longer life expectancies than those in developed countries without universal healthcare, according to a 2018 report published in Frontiers in Pharmacology.

Cultural problems may have an effect on one's health. A society's beliefs and rituals, as well as a family's reaction to them, may have a positive or negative effect on health.

According to the Seven Countries Study, researchers looked at people in a number of European countries and discovered that those who consumed a healthy diet had a lower death rate after 20 years.

People who ate a healthy diet were more likely to eat a lot of fruits, vegetables, and olives than people who ate fast food on a regular basis, according to the report.

People who consumed a Mediterranean diet had a lower 10-year all-cause mortality rate, according to the report. This diet, according to the International Journal of Environmental Research and Public Health, will help protect a person's heart and lower the risk of a variety of diseases, including type 2 diabetes, cancer, and diseases of the brain and nerves.

The way a person treats stress has an effect on their well-being. People who use tobacco, alcohol or illegal drugs to cope with stressful conditions are more likely to experience health issues, according to the National Institute of Mental Health, than those who use a balanced diet, coping methods, and exercise to cope.

~EMOTIONAL HEALTH~

Emotional health is critical to physical wellbeing. Emotionally stable people have power over their emotions, feelings, and behavior. They are capable of dealing with life's difficulties. They have the ability to keep problems in perspective and recover from setbacks. They are confident in themselves and in their relationships.

Being emotionally stable does not imply that you are always happy. It implies that you are conscious of your feelings. If they're positive or bad, you should work with them. People who are emotionally stable can experience tension, frustration, and sadness. They do, however, know how to deal with their negative emotions. They can tell when a problem is too big for them to tackle alone. They even know when to seek medical assistance.

Emotional wellbeing is an ability, according to research. You should take action to boost your mental wellbeing and happiness.

A path to better health

- ✓ Emotional wellbeing helps you to work effectively and deal with the pressures of daily life. It has the ability to assist you in realizing your full potential. It enables you to collaborate with others and contribute to society.
- ✓ It also has an effect on your physical well-being. There is a correlation between a positive mental attitude and physical signs of good health, according to studies. Lower pressure of the blood, a lower risk of heart disease, and a healthy weight are just a few of the benefits.
- ✓ There are several approaches to enhancing or maintaining mental wellbeing.
- ✓ Be conscious of your feelings and reactions.
- ✓ Take note of what makes you sad, irritated, or angry in your life. Make an attempt to fix or alter certain problems.
- ✓ Feelings should be expressed in acceptable ways.
- ✓ When anything bothers you, let anyone close to you know. Holding depression or frustration inside adds to the stress level. It can trigger issues in your personal life, as well as at work or school.
- ✓ Consider your options before taking action.
- ✓ Allow yourself time to reflect and relax before saying or doing anything you can come to regret.

- ✓ Take control of your pressures.
- ✓ To deal with tension, learn relaxation techniques. Deep breathing, meditation, and exercise are examples of these.
- ✓ Strive for equilibrium.
- ✓ Find a healthy balance between work and play, as well as physical activity and rest. Make time for the activities you love. Concentrate on the positive areas of your life.
- ✓ Take good care of your physical wellbeing.
- ✓ Get enough sleep, exercise, and eat nutritious meals. Do not use drugs or drink so much alcohol. Keep your physical well-being from impacting your mental well-being.
- ✓ Make friends with others.
- ✓ Make a lunch date, join a club, and say hello to people you don't know. We need meaningful interpersonal relations.
- ✓ Find sense and intent in your life.
- ✓ Determine what's most important to you in life and concentrate on it. This could be your career, family, voluntary work, caregiving, or something else entirely. Spend time doing stuff that matter to you.
- ✓ Maintain a good attitude.
- ✓ Concentrate on the positive aspects of your life. Forgive yourself and others for making mistakes.
- ✓ Spend time with people who are safe and optimistic.
- ✓ Although people with strong emotional health may suffer from emotional issues or mental illness. Mental disorder is often accompanied by physical symptoms. It's likely that

this is due to a chemical imbalance in the brain. Stress and problems with family, work, or school can either cause or worsen mental illness.

- ✓ People with emotional problems or mental illnesses may benefit from counseling, support groups, and medications. Consult your doctor if you have a chronic emotional issue. He or she may assist you in finding the necessary care.

~SPIRITUAL HEALTH~

What does it mean to be spiritually healthy?

Spirit is that which cannot be categorized as a part of the body or the mind. The effects of the body, mind, and spirit are all intertwined. You will help the healing process by strengthening your spiritual life. While spirituality cannot heal you, it can help you cope with the pain and difficulties that come with illness. When you are at peace with life, you are spiritually well. It's when you can find hope and comfort even in the most trying of circumstances. It may be able to assist you in fully experiencing life. Everyone's spirituality is special.

It's possible to lose your spiritual health when you're dealing with a chronic illness. There'll come a time when you'll be tempted to abandon your convictions. It's important to note that living a spiritually balanced life will help you maintain your physical health. Your spiritual life will assist you in coping with any physical health problems that might occur. We are complete individuals. Balance will help us stay safe and recover.

If you're having problems with your spiritual wellbeing, consider the following questions:

What makes me feel the most fulfilled?

When do I feel the most like I'm part of the rest of the world?

Where do I draw the most power from within?

What do I do when I'm feeling complete?

These questions can assist you in deciding what you can do to achieve inner peace. You will give your body more power for healing if you can find inner peace. Our physical bodies need that we be at ease.

This gives them the opportunity to relax and heal.

This is yet another way in which our spiritual wellbeing will aid our recovery.

~FINANCIAL HEALTH~

You are more than your bank account balance, but your financial situation may have an effect on other aspects of your life. When it comes to your general health, your finances should not be the first thing that comes to mind. However, studies show that your finances—not how much you have, but how you handle it—have an effect on your overall health and satisfaction. Living within your means, planning for emergencies and the future, and making informed choices about the resources you already have are all important aspects of financial health.

Financial wellbeing gives you peace of mind regarding your present and future investments. If you're in good financial shape, you're probably not concerned about money. You will likely have a monthly spending, investment, and savings strategy in place. If you're having financial difficulties, you might avoid discussing them with anyone, including your partner. If you've trouble controlling your spending and don't have a budget or schedule, you can be worried about finances, depressed, and have trouble sleeping.

Some aspects of your wellbeing are influenced by your financial situation:

- ***Relationships and money**:* Holding safe, open discussions about money and setting goals together can be beneficial to your relationship.
- ***Environment and finances**:* Making a meal plan will help you cut down on fast food and the plastic and packaging that comes with it.
- ***Finances and emotions**:* Individuals who are in control of their finances have fewer depressive episodes.
- ***Boosting your financial condition:*** Money can be intimidating at times, but beginning with one small habit at

a time might be all you need to change your situation and have a positive effect on your overall health and happiness.

Three things you need to do right now to change your financial situation:

- ***Compare:*** Look for the best price. Inculcate the habit of comparing prices and check for bargains before making a purchase.
- ***Financial planning:***Make a financial plan. Make it a routine to set a monthly budget and stick to it.
- ***Start putting money aside now!*** Open a savings account at your bank and set up an automatic monthly transfer if you don't already have one.

Financial health is important, but it's just one aspect of your overall heal.

PART II

~EATING HABITS YOU NEED TO APPLY~

You're not alone if you've vowed to become healthier and develop better eating habits in the new year. Although there are several different types of New Year's resolutions, many of us sit down in December and decide that this is the year we will genuinely commit to eating healthy and smarter. Finally, we're going to cut back on sugar, master portion control, consume more fruits and vegetables, and avoid eating a pint of ice cream right before bed. Even if you mean it, if you don't have a solid plan and strategy in place, your resolutions are likely to fail.

Healthy eating habits are well worth the effort. They'll hang with you all year, rather than vanishing in the middle of February like half the gymgoers. Susan Albers, Psy.D., a clinical psychologist at the Cleveland Clinic and a mindful eating specialist, tells SELF that the cornerstone of success is cultivating healthier and truly safe behaviors. "We love habits because we don't have to think about them," Albers says. "It doesn't seem like work at all."

"Putting a Band-Aid on a fractured arm is like putting a Band-Aid on a broken arm."
You are on the right foot if you approach January with the mentality that a habit shift, not just a crash diet, will help you lose weight quickly.

Here are some pretty easy changes you can make to your eating habits to help you achieve your target faster:

1. Ingest the rainbow

The color of every fruit and veggie is determined by the minerals, vitamins, phytochemicals, and antioxidants it contains. The more colors you use to paint your plate, the more nutrient variety you'll get. Furthermore, it keeps things exciting so that you do not get bored.

2. Experiment with new foods

We appear to eat the same things repeatedly. This restricts our food options. Try new stuff. Experiment with new foods. You could just find a new favorite that you've been missing out on.

3. Pay attention to what you're eating

According to Albers, mindful eating entails paying more attention to how you eat and being more present in order to make healthier food choices. She compares it to laying a stable base for a home. "If you master mindful feeding, it will be much easier to form new habits." Ignore all distractions and pay close attention to what you're putting on your plate and in your mouth instead of eating in front of the T.V. or screen. You'll be more relaxed, stop eating when you're fully satisfied, and make healthy decisions as a result.

4. Slow down when eating

Albers advises pausing before taking a bite and chewing slowly and carefully. This will assist you in refocusing your attention on the task at hand (eating) and keeping you from mindlessly scarfing down much more than your body requires.

5. Develop your stress management skills

Many people, according to Albers, have a poor habit of stress feeding. You'll eventually avoid turning to food for comfort if you find other ways to cope with stress. Find something other than food to help you unload your tension, whether it's reading a good book, having a manicure, cooking, going for a run, or whatever else helps you unwind and regroup.

6. Pay attention to the ingredient labels

If you don't know what's in the food you're eating, you'll never be able to cut down on added sugar or consume less sodium—or whatever other healthy-eating goal you have. We will find a lot of needless ingredients in the packaged foods we purchase at the grocery store. Jackie Baumrind, M.S., C.D.N., a dietitian at Selvera Wellness, recommends purchasing foods with a shorter ingredient list so you can consume the nutrients contained naturally in foods, which is a safe way to remain within healthy fat, carb, and sugar limits.

7. Cook more

What's the easiest way to find out what's in your food? You should make it yourself. You will also help manage portion sizes if you serve yourself—"If you serve yourself, you prefer to eat less," Baumrind tells SELF. She recommends experimenting with spices to make flavorful dishes with less sugar and salt than you would find in a restaurant.

8. Create a schedule

Albers notes, "This way, you click into doing it even though you don't feel like it." Eat at the same period every day, or set aside Sunday mornings to prepare meals. It will become second nature once it has become normal.

9. Make a kitchen reorganization

"Keep treats hidden and off the table. Albers recommends putting a fruit bowl on the counter. A "mindful makeover" will help you avoid cravings and allow you to really understand what your body wants and needs.

10. Never allow yourself to go hungry

We're all familiar with the scenario. We get caught up in work, kids, or whatever else is keeping us occupied, and before we know it, it's 3 p.m., and you haven't eaten since 8 a.m. Since our minds are telling us to feed, we give in to unhealthy cravings or binge on more than we need while we're ravenous. You will avoid this by planning out your meals and snacks during the day.

11. Have the measuring cups ready

Most of us have trouble with portion control, and it's mostly by mistake. We simply don't know what a proper portion size is. "Set aside some time on Sunday to break out the measuring cups," Baumrind advises. "Just have a general understanding of what a portion size is so that the eyes, stomach, and brain are all on the same page." When you're familiar with how objects appear, you'll be able to judge them more correctly at restaurants and holiday parties.

12. Use plates that are smaller

Another way to keep the portion sizes under control? Just use smaller plates. "There's no reason you have to use a 10-inch plate for a main course—you can use a salad plate," Baumrind says. "Use the larger plate for fruits and vegetables or salad at a holiday party, and the smaller plate for starches and protein." You'll be able to get closer to the right amount of each food without having to break out the measuring cups in the middle of the crowd (not recommended).

13. Increase the water intake

It's vital to stay hydrated throughout the day, not just when it's hot outside or you're working out at the gym. "We forget that when it's cold," Baumrind says. "Make sure you're having enough water" by using tricks like holding a water bottle at your desk or monitoring how much you're drinking with an app.

If you drink lots of sugary drinks, consider switching to unsweetened seltzer water (if you like bubbles) or fruit-infused water instead (hey, sugar fiend).

14. Start with the vegetables

"When my clients sit down for lunch or dinner, I try to get them to start with salad or vegetables and then dig into the rest," Baumrind says. She states that chewing lettuce and vegetables "pulls you through the moment, so you're not mindlessly eating." Plus, it is always a great idea to start with the healthiest foods.

15. Keep leftovers in the fridge

Make enough food for an extra meal or two so you can store leftovers in the fridge. This way, when you're hungry and short of time, you can turn to them instead of fast food.

16. Prepare snacks and meals

Meal preparation has many advantages, including eating better and saving money. Preparing snacks is also essential, according to Baumrind. "You should have a general idea of what snacks you want and should bring with you," she advises. "If you make a snack schedule ahead of time, you are more likely to snack and make healthier snack decisions."

17. Before you go, read the menu

If you eat out often, Baumrind recommends reading menus before going to a restaurant so you can walk in with a game plan. Same goes for holiday parties: make a mental list of which foods you'll prioritize and which you can skip (i.e., the foods you don't really like yet consume because they're traditional party fare). "You won't be fine, but you'll be better than if you show up without a strategy."

18. Make a half-sitting gesture

"We don't normally have an appetizer and a full main course at home," Baumrind explains. So you should do the same when you go out to eat. Split an appetizer with a friend, or split an entree and an appetizer with a friend so you could try more than one thing that sounds interesting. Sharing a meal often forces you to eat more mindfully, or you risk being the one who takes all the good stuff.

19. Don't be too hard on yourself when it comes to food

Eating is supposed to be a pleasurable experience. You're refueling your body and, hopefully, enjoying the process. Do you want to try that cookie? Consume the cookie! That cookie is fantastic!

Enjoy it, and you'll be happy you did. Focusing too much on eating "right" can lead to obsessing, as opposed to paying attention. Healthy eating, like so much else in life, is just about finding the right balance.

CHAPTER 4

~HEALTHY EATING: A SOURCE OF ENERGY~

Healthy eating is a way of managing the food intake in order to maintain good health. You'll have more energy during the day, get the vitamins and minerals you need, remain strong for the things you love, and maintain a healthy weight if you eat well.

QUESTION:

- ✓ Do you set aside time for breakfast?
- ✓ Are you able to go more than 4 hours without eating?
- ✓ Is dinner your key meal of the day?
- ✓ Do you prefer coffee, juice, or soda to water?
- ✓ Do you have a favorite vegetable that is a french fry?
- ✓ Do you spend the majority of your day at your desk, with no time to exercise?
- ✓ What are the 5 Most Significant Health Benefits of a Balanced Diet?

A Healthy Diet will help you to:

- Manage a healthy weight;
- Control blood sugar, blood cholesterol, and blood pressure ;

- Lower risk of chronic disease;
- Enhance immune system;
- Control appetite & food cravings;
- Increase energy & concentration;

ENERGY FROM FOOD

FOOD ENERGY

Food = Calories = Energy

Eat Digest Absorb Energy

Energy Yielding Nutrients: CARBOHYDRATES, PROTEIN, FAT

- ***CARBOHYDRATES (C.H.O.)***

✓ Body & brain's preferred source of energy;
✓ Converted into glucose in the body & raises blood sugar;
✓ Used for ENERGY;
✓ Stored as GLYCOGEN;
✓ Stored as F.A.T.;
✓ Three types: sugar, starch, fiber.

- ***CARBOHYDRATES***

✓ Sugar is the most essential form of carbohydrate;
✓ It's easily absorbed;
✓ It raises blood pressure quickly;
✓ It's quickly converted to glucose ENERGY (or stored).

- ***Fiber***

✓ Cannot be broken down;

✓ Does not increase blood sugar;

✓ Does not provide energy;

✓ Slows down sugar absorption gradual and steady rise in blood sugar longer lasting energy;

✓ Sugar: white and brown sugar, honey and syrup-apple, milk, and yogurt (natural).

- ***Starch***

✓ Bread, pasta, rice, cereal, oatmeal, starchy vegetables, beans, legumes, and starchy snack foods are all sources of starch (i.e., pretzels, chips).

- ***Fiber:*** whole grains, fruits, vegetables, beans, legumes, nuts, and seeds are all high in fiber.

- ***UNHEALTHY CARBS***

✓ Low in nutrients = "empty calories"- easily broken down and ingested - causes B.S. to spike high and then drop quickly;

✓ As a result, you'll have low energy and concentration, as well as exhaustion and hunger;

✓ White and brown sugar, butter, syrup, jam, juice, pop, and chocolate;

- ✓ Added sugar foods: baked goods, frozen sweets, granola bars, etc.;
- ✓ Refined Grains: white bread, rice, and pasta; low-fiber or sugary cereals (such as corn flakes); starchy snack foods.

- ***HEALTHY CARBS***
- ✓ Rich in nutrients;
- ✓ Take longer to digest and absorb;
- ✓ Cause a steady and moderate increase in B.S. and a smooth return to normal;
- ✓ As a result, more sustained energy and attention satiated and maximum appetite regulation;
- ✓ Whole grains: bread, crackers, and pasta are examples of whole grains; brown rice, cereal, and oatmeal are examples of whole grains.

- ***Starchy vegetables***
- ✓ Potatoes, yams, squash, corn, peas, beans/legumes (+ water, fiber);
- ✓ Fruit and Water-Based Vegetables (added water and fiber);
- ✓ Milk and yogurt (plus water and protein).

- ***PROTEIN***
- ✓ Used for muscle, tissue growth, and repair;
- ✓ Does not increase blood sugar;

- ✓ When combined with cholesterol, slows sugar absorption = longer-lasting energy and concentration.

- ***Healthy Proteins***
- ✓ Eggs, egg whites;
- ✓ Lean meat;
- ✓ White, skinless poultry;
- ✓ Fish, seafood;
- ✓ Beans, legumes;
- ✓ Nuts, seeds;
- ✓ Soy, tofu;
- ✓ Low fat milk, yogurt, cheese.

- ***F.A.T.***
- ✓ Not the brain's preferred energy source;
- ✓ Has no effect on blood sugar;
- ✓ Slows sugar absorption for longer;
- ✓ Lasting energy and concentration;
- ✓ "Healthy fat" is required in the diet, such as olive oil and grape seed oil. However, trans fat (found in many baked goods and fast foods) is not one of them.

- ***UNHEALTHY***
- ✓ Saturated fat;
- ✓ Butter, lard;
- ✓ Fat meats, poultry;

- ✓ Fat dairy: cream, cheese, ice cream;
- ✓ Tropical oils: coconut, palm.

- ***Trans fat***
- ✓ Hard margarine;
- ✓ Deep fried food;
- ✓ Muffins, pastry, doughnuts;
- ✓ Processed food: cookies, crackers.

- ***Healthy Fat***
- ✓ Oil:olive, grape seed, flaxseed;
- ✓ Salad Dressing (made with safe oil);
- ✓ Non-Hydrogenated Margarine, i.e., becel;
- ✓ Nuts, seeds;
- ✓ Nut or Seed Butter;
- ✓ Avocado;
- ✓ Low Fat Mayo, Sour Cream, Dairy.

Getting the proper quantity of protein, carbs, fiber, fat, and nutrients in the right mix at regular intervals in the day could help you maintain balanced blood sugar and energy levels.

- ***Boost your energy and concentration***
- ✓ Consume well-balanced meals and snacks;
- ✓ Watch the portion sizes;
- ✓ 3-4 hours between meals;

- ✓ Caffeine intake should be restricted;
- ✓ Drink plenty of water and keep involved.

- ***Balanced meals and snacks***
- ✓ Adequate protein, carbohydrates (C.H.O.), fiber, and healthy fat;
- ✓ Calorie, fat, and sugar content are all low (fruits and vegetables);
- ✓ Carbohydrates that are complex–peptide (beans, fish, chicken, tofu).

- ***Achieving Balance***
- ✓ Choosing foods from:at least three to four meal groups + two groups of SNACKS = "Balanced, Healthy Eating" with all nutrients!

- ***PORTION CONTROL HELPS PREVENT***
- ✓ High and low blood sugar and energy ;
- ✓ Fatigue and lethargy ;
- ✓ Feeling of fullness ;
- ✓ Weight gain.

- ***TIPS FOR PORTION CONTROL***
- ✓ Portion out your food before consuming it - don't eat out of bags or containers;
- ✓ Use small cups, dishes, and utensils when dining out ;

- ✓ Ask for dips, dressings, sauces, and spreads on the side when eating out ;
- ✓ Load up on vegetables to fill you up!
- ***EAT FREQUENTLY***
- ✓ Prevents blood sugar lows;
- ✓ Provides a steady supply of calories for the body and brain;
- ✓ Maintains energy and attention levels.

- ✓ ***DRINK WATER***
- ✓ Prevents appetite and desires to overeat later in the day;
- ✓ Most foods count – fruit, vegetables, dairy;
- ✓ 8-9 cups a day (individual variability);
- ✓ Needs – salt, sugar, caffeine, alcohol, exercise, heat;
- ✓ Dehydration induces fatigue, low energy, and weak concentration.

CHAPTER 5

~WHAT TO EAT TO HAVE A HEALTHY LIFESTYLE?~

"What is a healthy diet?"

Many clinicians are stumped when it comes to responding to this common query from patients. It's understandable that providing a straightforward response is difficult. The vast amount of data generated by food and nutrition researchers, combined with sometimes contradictory findings, apparent flip-flops in recommendations, and a flood of misinformation in diet books and the media, can make it seem as if explaining the basics of healthy eating is akin to explaining particle physics. That's a shame because there are now enough strong strands of evidence from reputable sources to weave clear but convincing dietary guidelines.

The average woman in the U.S. and other developed countries can expect to live for 80 years or more.
With such longevity, simply consuming the calories required to maintain, create, and rebuild the body isn't enough. Chronic diseases like heart disease, cancer, osteoporosis, and age-related vision loss can all be influenced by the foods that provide these calories. While there's still much to learn on the importance of

specific nutrients in reducing the risk of chronic disease, a broad body of evidence suggests that balanced dietary habits that prioritize whole grains, legumes, vegetables, and fruits while limiting refined starches, red meat, full-fat dairy products, and foods and beverages high in added sugars are beneficial. Diets like these have been linked to a lower risk of a number of chronic diseases.

Of course, diet is only one method for avoiding illness. Other effective techniques include reducing food intake to maintain a healthy weight, exercising regularly, and not smoking. The Nurses' Health Research showed that women who adopted a healthy lifestyle pattern that included these four interventions were 80 percent less likely than all other women in the study to experience cardiovascular disease over a 14-year period. Men, too, benefited from similar healthier decisions, according to a companion report, the Health Professionals Follow-up Study, even though they were taking blood pressure or cholesterol-lowering drugs.

FAT IN THE DIET

Dietary fat is a nutrient that is commonly overlooked and unfairly maligned. Fat is evil, according to myths and messages that have existed since the 1960s. This risky oversimplification has aided the production of thousands of fat-free yet calorie-dense foods, as well as hundreds of relatively unsuccessful diets.

It has also contributed to the obesity and type 2 diabetes epidemics. Since there are four major types of dietary fat, each with significantly different health consequences, the message "fat is evil" is problematic. Trans fats derived from partially hydrogenated oils are unquestionably harmful to the heart and the rest of the body. These mostly man-made fats raise harmful low-density lipoprotein (LDL) cholesterol, lower protective high-density lipoprotein (HDL) cholesterol, induce inflammation and a number of other changes that damage arteries and impair cardiovascular health.

Trans fat consumption has been linked to an increased risk of cardiovascular disease, type 2 diabetes, gallstones, dementia, and weight gain.

Saturated fats from red meat and dairy products raise LDL cholesterol while also raising HDL. Saturated fat consumption in moderation (less than 8% of daily calories) is consistent with a balanced diet, although higher levels have been linked to cardiovascular disease. Monounsaturated and polyunsaturated fats, especially polyunsaturated omega-3 fatty acids, found in vegetable oils, seeds, nuts, whole grains, and fish, are important components of a balanced diet and essential for cardiac health. Polyunsaturated fats replace saturated and trans fats in the diet, which reduces dangerous LDL, increases protective HDL, enhances insulin sensitivity, and stabilizes heart rhythms. Dietary fat isn't related to a higher risk of chronic disease. In fact, diets of up to 40% fat calories can be very safe if they are low in trans and also saturated fat but high in polyunsaturated and monounsaturated fat. While conclusive evidence on the ideal dietary fat proportions is missing, a low trans and saturated fat intake and a higher unsaturated fat intake minimize the risk of cardiovascular disease and diabetes.

CARBOHYDRATES

In the United States, the decline in dietary fat consumption from 45 percent of calories in 1965 to about 34 percent today was followed by a rise in carbohydrate consumption. The majority of the extra carbohydrates came from highly processed grains. Processed grains, such as white flour or white rice, lose fiber, healthy fats, and a variety of vitamins, minerals, and phytonutrients, rendering them nutritionally deficient in comparison to whole-grain varieties. A diet high in highly processed grains is linked to a rise in triglycerides and a decrease in protective HDL cholesterol. These negative reactions can be exacerbated by insulin resistance, which commonly develops during pregnancy. Insulin resistance and type 2 diabetes are on the rise in the United States and around the world.

The Glycemic Index (G.I.)

The glycemic reaction is the observable rise in blood sugar that occurs after eating carbohydrates. The higher the postprandial spike in glucose that a food causes, the higher its glycemic index.

As compared to less processed whole grains, highly refined grains induce a faster and larger overall rise in blood sugar. Increased plasma insulin levels follow higher glycemic responses, which are thought to be at the root of metabolic syndrome and have also been related to ovulatory infertility.

Diets high in glycemic index or glycemic load (the result of dietary glycemic index and total carbohydrate intake) tend to increase the risk of type 2 diabetes and coronary artery disease, especially in women with insulin resistance. The milling process causes a substantial loss of fiber and micronutrients, which may lead to the negative effects of highly processed grains. Whole grains, whole-grain foods, fruits, vegetables, and beans, on the other hand, have slowly digested carbohydrates, which are high in fiber, vitamins, minerals, and phytonutrients. A large body of evidence suggests that consuming whole grains or high-fiber cereals instead of highly processed grains lowers the risk of cardiovascular disease and type 2 diabetes. While it has been difficult to prove that diets high in whole-grain fiber reduce the risk of colon cancer, such a dietary pattern has been linked to a reduction in constipation and diverticular disease.

PROTEIN

It makes no difference if amino acids come from animal or plant protein to metabolic processes involved in protein development and repair. Protein, on the other hand, is not eaten in isolation.

Instead, it comes in a box with a range of other vitamins and minerals. Long-term health can be influenced by the quality and amount of fats, carbohydrates, sodium, and other nutrients in the "protein kit." The Nurses' Health Study, for instance, found that eating more protein from beans, nuts, seeds, and other sources while limiting easily digested carbohydrates lowers the risk of heart disease. 16 In that research, consuming more animal protein while decreasing carbohydrate intake did not reduce the risk of heart disease, likely due to the fats and other nutrients that come (or do not come) with animal protein.

FRUITS AND VEGETABLES

"Eat more fruits and vegetables" is advice that has stood the test of time and is backed by a wide body of evidence. Fiber, slowly digested carbohydrates, vitamins and minerals, and various phytonutrients found in vegetables and fruits have been linked to defense against cardiovascular disease, aging-related vision loss due to cataract and macular degeneration, and bowel function maintenance. The connection between fruits, vegetables, and cancer is less well understood. Fruits and vegetables, while not having a universal anticancer effect, can help with specific cancers such as esophageal, stomach, lung, and colorectal cancer. Fruits and veggies should be eaten in large quantities, with at least five servings a day recommended—more is better. In the United States, only about one out of every four people meets this requirement.

BEVERAGES

The perfect beverage contains 100% of what the body requires—H2O—and contains no calories or additives. Water meets all of these requirements. It costs a part of a penny per glass if you have it straight from the bottle. Tea and coffee are most widely consumed drinks after water. Both are relatively healthy drinks that have been related to a lower risk of type 2 diabetes, kidney stones, gallstones, heart failure, and some forms of cancer.

Sugar-sweetened beverages (sodas, fruit drinks, juices, sports drinks, and so on) and alcoholic beverages are two of the most troublesome beverages. A 12-ounce can of sugar-sweetened cola contains 8–10 teaspoons of sugar or about 120–150 calories of "empty" calories. Consumption of sugary drinks on a daily basis has been linked to weight gain and an increased risk of type two diabetes, disease of the heart, and gout.

Moderate alcohol consumption (no more than one drink per day for women, 1–2 drinks per day for men) has been linked to lower cardiovascular disease and type 2 diabetes risks. Moderate drinking, on the other hand, can increase the risk of breast cancer. A diet high in folate, on the other hand, can help to reduce this risk.

Drinking alcohol during pregnancy is not advised due to the possible health hazards to the unborn child.

MINERALS AND VITAMINS

Vitamins, minerals, and other micronutrients required for good health are commonly found in an optimal diet. However, many women in the United States, including a significant number of disadvantaged women, do not eat optimally. As a result, for the majority of women, a daily multivitamin-multimineral supplement is adequate protection against nutritional deficiencies. Extra iron is typically included in these supplements and is needed by the 9 percent to 11 percent of premenopausal women who are iron deficient. The most well-documented advantage of vitamin supplements is that extra folic acid can reduce the risk of neural tube defects by about 70%.

Calcium is essential for bone strength to be maintained. The exact amount of calcium required is a contentious topic. The World Health Organization recommends an intake of 400 mg daily. For women aged 19 and up, 700 mg per day is considered sufficient in the United Kingdom. Adult women in the United States can consume 1,500 mg of calcium a day, which can be obtained in large part by consuming three servings of low-fat or fat-free dairy products a day. Calcium supplements are a low-calorie and fat-free alternative.

Other factors, such as physical activity and vitamin D, are just as important as calcium in preserving bone strength. There is mounting evidence that current vitamin D guidelines (200–600 IU/day, depending on age) are too poor and that 1,000 IU/day protects against fractures, heart disease, and some cancers. Excess

preformed vitamin A consumption has been linked to an increased risk of hip fracture, likely due to vitamin D competition.
However, intakes slightly higher than the current Dietary Reference Intake of 700 g per day are associated with an increased risk. Given this issue, a multivitamin that provides a significant amount of vitamin A in the form of beta-carotene is favored.

EXERCISE AND WEIGHT CONTROL

The core of a web of health and illness is a spider's web of body weight. Excess weight puts an individual at risk of developing a number of chronic illnesses. The greater the incidence of elevated blood glucose, lipids, and blood pressure; hypertension and cardiovascular disease; diabetes; many cancers; gallstones; sleep apnea; pregnancy complications; infertility; and premature mortality, the higher the B.M.I.> 25 kg/m2.

According to current national guidelines, a B.M.I. of 18 to 25 kg/m2 is considered ideal, and the best health is obtained by preventing weight gain during adulthood.
Calories ingested and spent play a direct role in maintaining a healthy body weight or losing weight.

Weight maintenance necessitates portion management. Low consumption of sugary drinks and trans fats, as well as a higher intake of dietary fiber, tend to be beneficial when it comes to weight maintenance. Regular exercise and avoiding extreme inactivity, such as excessive television consumption, are both effective weight-control techniques. It's also necessary to have a positive social and physical atmosphere.

PATTERNS IN DIET

While research on fats, carbohydrates, and specific vitamins and minerals has been successful, it has also led to some dead ends, as well as misconceptions and misunderstandings on what constitutes healthy eating. People consume food rather than nutrients, which is one of the main reasons. Furthermore, humans have reasonably consistent dietary habits. Although studying dietary patterns is more difficult than studying nutrients, recent research has shown that certain dietary patterns are beneficial to long-term health. The traditional Western diet, which's high in red meat, highly refined grains, and sugar and low in fruits, vegetables, whole grains, and fiber, is one dietary pattern that can affect long-term health. This form of dietary pattern has been linked to atherosclerosis and a number of cardiovascular disorders; heart attack and stroke, peripheral artery disease, and heart failure, according to numerous reports.

The Department of Health and Human Services is also a part of the process as well. The guidelines "provide authoritative guidance for people two years and older on how healthy dietary habits can improve health and minimize risk for major chronic diseases," according to the USDA.

The Food Guide Pyramid was created in an attempt to make the instructions more available to the general public. Regrettably, this iconic emblem reflected the aims of American agriculture as well as the ideals of healthy eating. The Food Guide Pyramid didn't mention grains; instead, it lumped red meat, poultry, fish, and beans together and instructed us to measure them by their total fat content. The Food Guide Pyramid encouraged people to drink three glasses of low-fat milk or eat three servings of other dairy products every day and made no distinction between different forms of fat, advising people to consume fat "sparingly." The Food Guide Pyramid was replaced in the year 2005 by the MyPyramid, which can only be deciphered using the MyPyramid Web site. The food industry praised the use of vertical stripes to replace food groups since the original Food Guide Pyramid depicted foods near the bottom as "healthy" and those near the top as "evil." All foods are nutritionally identical in the left-to-right style.

A better dietary pattern is represented by the Healthy Eating Pyramid, which was developed by Harvard School of Public Health faculty members based on the best available evidence.

For people who would rather adopt a set dietary plan than create their own based on the Balanced Eating Pyramid, a Mediterranean-style diet or the DASH diet can have significant health benefits.

Dietary Guidelines for the Mediterranean

Orthodox Mediterranean diets have been related to lower rates of heart disease and other chronic diseases in countries surrounding the Mediterranean Sea. Such diets also tend to adapt well to new environments. The 166,012 women who took part in the National Institutes of Health AARP Diet and Health Study had lower risks of all-cause mortality (multivariate hazard ratio [H.R.], 0.80; 95 percent confidence interval [CI], 0.75–0.85), cardiovascular mortality (H.R., 0.81; 95 percent CI, 0.68–0.97), and cancer mortality (H.R., 0.88; 95 percent CI, 0.78–1.00).

For men, there was a similar pattern. The effect was even more pronounced in smokers. Other health advantages of the Mediterranean diet include a lower risk of cancer, Parkinson's disease, and Alzheimer's disease. It has also been linked to asthma control36 and rheumatoid arthritis improvement. While no particular diet can be considered "the" Mediterranean diet, those that are deserving of the name have high extra virgin olive oil content, whole grains and fiber, and fruits, vegetables, legumes, and nuts. Tiny amounts of cheese and yogurt are eaten on a daily basis; fish is consumed in different amounts; red meat, poultry, eggs, and candy are consumed in moderation. Moderate quantities of red wine are consumed with meals, and daily physical exercise is encouraged.

WEIGHT LOSS AND DIET CONTROL

Almost any diet that lets the dieter eat fewer calories than she burns will result in weight loss, at least temporarily. Few dieters, on the other hand, are able to stick to weight-loss diets for long periods of time. No single diet is right for all due to variations in palates, food tastes, family circumstances, and even genes. A long-term dietary pattern that is good for the heart, bones, brain, psyche, and taste buds, as well as the waistline, is needed. There should be lots of variety in this diet, with few limits or "extra" foods.

According to randomized studies, the nutrient composition of a dietary pattern for weight loss is much less important than the number of calories it provides.

In a head-to-head analysis of four diets loosely based on the Atkins, Ornish, and Mediterranean diets, participants lost approximately 13.2 pounds (6 kg) and had a 2-inch drop in waist circumference. Most people started to recover weight after 12 months. Participants assigned to a diet with 25 percent protein and those assigned to a diet with 15 percent protein lost equal amounts of weight after two years (average of 4.5 and 3.6 kg, respectively; P=0.11), as did those assigned to a diet with 40 percent fat and those assigned to a diet with 20 percent fat (average of 3.9 and 4.1 kg, respectively; P=0.11). 58 Within the goal range of 35 percent to 65 percent of calories from carbohydrate, there was no impact of carbohydrate amount on weight loss.

The waist circumference changed in a similar way around the diet classes. Hunger, satiety, and diet satisfaction were consistent across the board, as were cholesterol levels and other cardiovascular risk markers. It's worth noting that these averages mask huge disparities in weight loss, with some participants losing 30 pounds or more and others gaining weight during the study. This backs up the idea that weight-loss plans should be tailored to the person.

Weight loss was supported by group therapy, meaning that physiological, psychological, and social factors are likely more important for weight loss than the dietary composition of a diet.

How to Make a Nutritional Grocery List

Even for the most organized individual, grocery shopping can be a challenging activity.
Every aisle seems to be brimming with enticing, unhealthy foods, threatening to derail your fitness goals.
A shopping list is a useful tool that will assist you in navigating the supermarket and sticking to your balanced eating schedule.
A well-planned shopping list will serve as a memory aid as well as keep you on track, reducing impulse purchases and saving you money. It will also help you thrive even if you are short on time by allowing you to have healthy food on hand to eat during the week.
Furthermore, studies have shown that shopping with a list results in healthy food decisions and even weight loss.

The following suggestions will assist you in creating a balanced grocery shopping list so that you can stock your cart with wise purchases.

Prepare ahead of time

Having the ingredients on hand to make delicious meals all week is a great way to stay on track with your diet.

When you have an empty fridge, freezer, or pantry, you can be tempted to eat fast food or order takeout, particularly if you have a busy schedule. That's why it's important to have a variety of healthy foods on hand.

People who prepare their meals ahead of time have a better overall diet and are less overweight than people who do not.

Plus, people who prepare their meals ahead of time are more likely to cook at home, which has been related to improved diet quality and lower body fat levels.

Making it a point to prepare your meals for the week will help you avoid making bad decisions and make a more effective grocery shopping list.

Making a recipe board with the recipes you want to eat for the week, including breakfasts, lunches, dinners, and snacks, is a great way to get started planning your meals.

Add the ingredients you'll need to make your meals to your shopping list after you've figured out what you'll need. Make sure to include the amount of each food you'll need.

Create a shopping list that is checked on a regular basis

Keep a list of the items you need to purchase on your next trip to the grocery store instead of trying to recall which favorite pantry staple you recently ran out of.

Keep track of your kitchen inventory with dry erase boards or magnetic to-do lists that hang on your fridge.

There are also several applications available to assist you with grocery shopping and meal preparation.

Keeping track of the foods you eat and the fresh and nutritious foods you want to try will make putting together your weekly shopping list much easier.

The first step in making a balanced grocery shopping list is to prepare your meals. Making a shopping list focused on pre-planned meals will assist you in preparing healthy dishes that adhere to your diet.

Be frank with yourself

It's crucial to be realistic about the foods you'll really eat while making a balanced shopping list.

When you first start eating more nutritiously, you might want to try a lot of new and different foods, but limit yourself to only a few new healthy foods each week.

It's easy to get distracted by things that appeal to you when you go grocery shopping without a list.

This could lead you to buy more food than you can reasonably consume in a week, or you may select foods that you can eat but don't really enjoy.

This can lead to squandered food and diminished financial resources.

Adding a few new foods to your meals each week is a great way to broaden your palate, add nutrients, and discover which nutritious foods you really enjoy.

If you want to eat more fresh, leafy vegetables like kale, arugula, and spinach but aren't sure which ones to try, try one new leafy green per week before you find a few favorites.

This will encourage you to try new foods without having to worry about wasting food or money.

You'll be able to make a new shopping list every week, full of nutritious foods you enjoy consuming before you know it.

When you're trying out new recipes, try adding one or two new ingredients every week to help you figure out which ones you really like. You can prevent wasting food and resources by gradually adding new foods.

Prepare Your To-Do List

Organizing your grocery shopping list by category is a smart way to save time and minimize stress on your trips to the supermarket.

You can sort your shopping list by food group or by the layout of your local grocery store.

Organizing your shopping list into parts allows you to shop more efficiently and reduces the likelihood of impulse purchases.

Instead of being overwhelmed by the countless unhealthy foods on the supermarket shelves, this type of list keeps you on track and focused on the things you've planned.

To begin, divide your list into parts based on the different types of foods. Vegetables, fruits, protein, carbohydrates, and healthy fats are among the categories.

• Dairy and non-dairy foods

• Condiments

• Drinks

Avoid making room on your shopping list for treats or desserts if you're trying to cut back on snacking or don't want to have candy in the house.

To keep your attention on wholesome, nutrient-dense foods, limit your list to only safe categories.

If you're familiar with your grocery store's layout, divide your list into parts based on the items you want to buy. List your fruits and vegetables first, for example, if you normally start your shopping trip in the produce aisle.

You'll be able to streamline your shopping trip and stop having to return to a certain section this way.

This reduces the risk of being tempted by unhealthy products when browsing the grocery store for foods on your shopping list.

Organizing your grocery shopping list into groups will help you stay focused, save time, and avoid making unhealthy decisions.

Place a focus on nutritious foods

When making your shopping list, aim to include foods that are nutritious and balanced.

This can be difficult, especially for those who have only recently begun a healthy eating plan.

Grocery shopping lists will help you avoid buying unhealthy items that will make you gain weight and sabotage your weight-loss efforts.

Before you go shopping, make sure your list is broken down into parts and includes everything you'll need to prepare healthy meals for the next few days.

If you know some parts of the grocery store, such as the bakery or the candy aisle, are especially tempting, it's a good idea to avoid them altogether.

Perimeter Shopping

Perimeter shopping helps you to concentrate on fresh foods while restricting your exposure to packaged and processed foods.

Fruits, vegetables, nutritious proteins, and dairy are commonly found around the perimeter of most supermarkets.

While there are many healthier choices in the interior supermarket aisles, such as canned and dried beans, grains, spices, and olive oil, most grocery chains also stock highly processed foods like candy, soda, and chips.

Spending less time in the grocery store's interior will reduce your exposure to unhealthy items, decreasing your risk of being tempted to buy them.

Since high-processed food consumption has been linked to obesity and chronic diseases such as heart disease and diabetes, limiting your intake is critical for maintaining your health and losing weight.

Filling your shopping list with mostly whole, unprocessed foods from the store's perimeter will help you include more nutritious foods in your diet.

Stick to your shopping list and concentrate on foods on the store's perimeter to avoid purchasing products that aren't good for you.

Stick to the plan

Whether it's for nutritious or unhealthy items, grocery stores are built to get customers to spend money. To stop temptation, go to the grocery store with a balanced eating plan in mind and just purchase the items on your list.

Advertisements in stores and weekly flyers advertising coupons and discounts can have a big influence on the foods you buy.

Unfortunately, some grocery stores' promotions focus on processed goods rather than fresh produce.

That's one of the reasons it's crucial to begin your shopping trip with a well-thought-out shopping list. Sticking to your list will help you avoid making impulsive purchases of unhealthy foods or products you won't use just because they're on sale.

However, eye-catching shows and deep discounts make it all too easy to get distracted.

Take the time to consider whether a sale item or a fancy food display fits into your meal plan and to remind yourself of your balanced shopping list if you are drawn in by a sale item or a fancy food display.

Making a nutritious and delicious grocery list ahead of time and committing to buy only the items on it will help you stay on track with your balanced eating plan and avoid being swayed by commercials and sales.

To Get You Started, These Are Some Healthy Examples

It's best to prioritize new, whole foods while making your shopping list.

Though it's perfectly natural and safe to have a treat now and then, keep candy and snack foods to a minimum while making your shopping list.

Excessive consumption of highly processed foods such as sugary cereals, candy, soda, chips, and baked goods will sabotage your weight loss attempts and cause you to gain weight.

Here are a few examples of good, nutritious foods that you can add to your shopping cart.

- ***Non-starchy vegetables:*** broccoli, beets, cauliflower, asparagus, onions, carrots, bell peppers, spinach, kale, arugula, mixed greens, radishes, green beans, zucchini, tomatoes, Brussels sprouts, mushrooms, broccoli, beets, cauliflower, asparagus, onions, carrots, bell peppers, spinach, kale, arugula, mixed greens, radishes, green beans, zucchini, tomatoes, Brussels sprouts, mushrooms;

- ***Fruits:*** berries, bananas, apples, grapes, grapefruit, oranges, lemons, limes, pears, cherries, pineapple, pomegranate, kiwis, and mangoes are among the fruits accessible;
- ***Proteins:*** eggs, shrimp, pork, chicken, fresh turkey breast, tofu, bison, and beef are all healthy sources of protein;
- ***Carbohydrates:*** sweet potatoes, potatoes, oats, butternut squash, quinoa, brown rice, beans, lentils, chia seeds, buckwheat, barley, and whole-grain bread are all good sources of carbohydrates;
- ***Healthy fats:*** olives, olive oil, avocados, avocado oil, coconut, coconut oil, almonds, seeds, almond butter, peanut butter, cashew butter, tahini, pesto, ground flaxseeds are all good sources of healthy fats;
- ***Dairy and Non Dairy products***: greek yogurt, butter, cottage cheese, almond milk, coconut milk, goat cheese, kefir, and unsweetened milk are examples of dairy and non-dairy products;
- ***Condiments***: salsa, apple cider vinegar, balsamic vinegar, spices, herbs, stone-ground mustard, horseradish,

nutritional yeast, sauerkraut, hot sauce, raw honey, and stevia.

- ***Drinks:*** sparkling water, unsweetened seltzer, green tea, coffee, ginger tea, unsweetened iced tea.

These are a few of the many nutritious and delicious items you can have on your shopping list.

Organize your shopping list by what makes the most sense to you to make it easier to shop.

Avocado, for example, is actually a fruit, but most people think of it as a tasty source of healthy fat.

Whatever tool you use to build your shopping list, make sure it is well-organized and simple to read so you can enjoy a stress-free shopping experience.

A nutritious grocery list should include a range of healthy foods. Increasing your intake of mostly whole, unprocessed foods will help you become healthier and achieve your nutritional goals.

Shopping for groceries doesn't have to be difficult.

Using a shopping list to drive you around the supermarket is a perfect way to keep on board with your diet goals.

In addition, making a meal plan and shopping list ahead of time will save you time and money.

Making a balanced grocery shopping list should be at the top of your to-do list, given the possible benefits.

SAMPLE OF A HEALTHY SHOPPING LIST

We should all agree that if you don't go to the grocery store with a strong list, you'll end up spending a lot of money.

The best way for good health is to consume more whole, nutrient-dense foods and avoid processed foods as much as possible.

Vegetables

- spinach
- arugula
- kale
- broccoli
- cauliflower
- bell peppers
- brussels sprouts
- zucchini
- carrots
- asparagus
- cabbage
- cucumbers
- celery
- onions
- garlic
- new herbs including basil and parsley
- potatoes and sweet potatoes

Fruits

• avocados (at varying stages of ripeness)

•fresh blueberries, strawberries, blackberries, or raspberries (buy frozen to save money)

• apples

• oranges, lemons, limes, and grapefruit

• pomegranate

• grapes (green or red)

• bananas

• pineapple

• cherries

Dairy products

• pasture butter

• eggs (preferably pasture-raised)

• full-fat grass-fed yogurt, 2% yogurt, or coconut yogurt

• coconut milk, almond milk, or dairy milk (unsweetened, nondairy milks that contain limited ingredients)

• full-fat cheeses like goat, cheddar, and feta; sauerkraut, kimchi, and kefir

Meat, fish, and vegetarian proteins

• whole chicken or skinless chicken breasts (use it all in the soup!)

• wild caught salmon in a can (hint: almost all canned salmon is wild-caught!)

• shell fish such as shrimp or crab

• new fish fillets such as flounder or cod

• vegetarian protein sources like extra-firm tofu or tempeh

• ground turkey or grass-fed beef or pork

Grain and legume goods

• quinoa, amaranth, brown rice, teff, farro, buckwheat, barley, and millet • grains such as quinoa, amaranth, brown rice, teff, farro, buckwheat, barley, and millet (Find them in individual packages or in the bulk food section of some grocery stores)

• rolled or steel-cut oats (Skip the sugary instant oatmeal and go for plain rolled or steel-cut oats with your own toppings instead)

• corn tortillas with just a few ingredients

Fruits and vegetables (Freezer staples)

• frozen greens, such as spinach and kale; frozen chopped vegetables, such as broccoli and cauliflower, edamame, and frozen fruits, such as grapes, cherries, cubed mango, and pomegranate seeds.

Bread and flour

Ezekiel bread, almond flour, coconut flour, wheat germ, and whole wheat flour.

Proteins

- frozen skin-on chicken breast
- frozen ground turkey

- frozen wild-caught fish and shellfish

Oils and fats

The following are some examples of healthy, minimally processed fats that can support your health in a number of ways:

- coconut oil
- tahini
- unsweetened coconut flakes and coconut butter
- olive oil
- avocado oil
- ghee or grass-fed butter

Nuts and butters

- almonds
- pumpkin seeds
- real peanut butter (only peanuts and salt)
- almond butter
- sunflower seeds
- chia seeds
- walnuts
- pistachios
- hemp seeds (These tiny seeds are filled with vitamins, minerals, and healthy fats.) They're great in smoothies, yogurt, and oatmeal, among other things.)
- Ground flaxseed

Condiments

- apple cider vinegar
- balsamic vinegar
- honey
- hot sauce
- pure maple syrup
- tamari, soy sauce, or coconut aminos
- nutritional yeast
- salsa
- mustard
- vanilla extract

Spices

Turmeric, ginger, cinnamon, sage, red pepper flakes, garlic powder, nutmeg, saffron, paprika, curry powder, and chili powder.

Canned goods

- full fat canned goods
- no-sugar-added marinara sauce
- coconut milk
- sardines
- crushed tomatoes
- pumpkin purée

Miscellaneous

• chicken broth
• baking powder
• baking soda
• cacao and cacao nibs
• sun-dried tomatoes

Beverage

• Teabags (green and black are great)
• peppermint, hibiscus, and ginger herbal teas
• sparkling water
• coffee

Snack foods

• dark chocolate
• grass-fed, nitrite- and sugar-free meat or turkey sticks or jerky
• pickles
• olives
• unsweetened dried fruits like raisins, figs, mango, or apple rings

CHAPTER 6

~HOW TO COMBINE FOODS CORRECTLY~

Food mixing is an eating philosophy of ancient origins that has recently gained a lot of attention.

Proper food combinations, according to proponents of food-combining diets, can lead to illness, toxin accumulation, and digestive distress.

They also agree that the right combinations will help to alleviate these issues.

Is there any validity in these statements, though?

What Is Food Combining?

The word "food mixing" refers to the notion that some foods complement each other while others do not.

It is assumed that mixing foods wrongly — for example, consuming steak with potatoes — may have negative health and digestive implications.

Food combining concepts first appeared in ancient India's Ayurvedic medicine, but they were popularized in the mid-nineteenth century as trophology, or "the science of food combining."

The Hay diet resurrected the ideals of food mixing in the early 1900s. They've been a staple of many western diets since then.

In general, food-combination diets divide foods into classes.

Carbohydrates and starches, fruits (including sweet fruits, acidic fruits, and melons), vegetables, proteins, and fats are the most common breakdowns.

Some plans, on the other hand, categorize foods as acidic, alkaline, or neutral.

Food-combination diets determine how these groups should be mixed in a meal.

Food Combination Rules

The laws of food pairing differ depending on the source, but the following are the most general guidelines:

- Avoid combining starches and proteins
- Eating fruit on an empty stomach, particularly melons.
- Don't mix starches and acidic foods
- Don't mix different types of protein
- Only eat dairy products, particularly milk, on an empty stomach.

Other tips include not combining protein with fat, only consuming sugar on its own, and eating fruits and vegetables separately.

Food Combining Is Based On Two Beliefs

The majority of food pairing laws are based on two beliefs.

The first is that when different foods digest at different rates, mixing a fast-digesting food with a slow-digesting food creates a "traffic jam" in your digestive tract, resulting in negative digestive and health effects.

The second belief is that different foods need different enzymes to break them down, and that these enzymes function in your gut at different pH levels (acidity levels).

The theory goes that if two foods need different pH levels, the body won't be able to digest them both at the same time.

Food-combining diet proponents agree that these values are critical to good health and digestion.

It's also thought that eating the wrong foods together has negative health effects including digestive discomfort, toxin development, and disease.

Food mixing is a form of eating in which various types of foods are not consumed at the same time. Proper food combinations, according to advocates of food-combining diets, lead to illness and digestive distress.

What Does the Proof Show?

Only one research has looked at the concepts of food pairing so far. It looked at whether a diet focused on food pairings helped people lose weight.

The participants were grouped into two and offered either a healthy diet or a diet based on food mixing principles.

They were only allowed to consume 1,100 calories per day on both diets.

Participants in both groups lost an average of 13–18 lbs (6–8 kg) after six weeks, but the food-combining diet had little advantage over the healthy diet.

In fact, most of the apparently scientific concepts of food pairing are unsupported by proof.

Many of the first food-combination diets were devised over a century ago, when nothing was understood about human nutrition and digestion.

However, much of the principles of food mixing are clearly contradicted by what we now know about basic biochemistry and nutritional science.

Let us have a clearer look at the science that backs up the arguments.

Why You Shouldn't Eat Mixed Meals

Meals that contain a mixture of fat, carbohydrates, and protein are referred to as "mixed meals."

The laws of food pairing are primarily based on the assumption that the human body is incapable of digesting mixed meals.

This, however, is obviously not true. Whole foods, which almost always contain a mixture of grains, protein, and fat, are what the human body developed on.

Vegetables and grains, for example, are commonly thought of as carbohydrate-rich foods. However, each serving contains several grams of protein. And, although meat is considered a protein-rich food, even lean meat contains fat.

Since several foods contain a mixture of carbohydrates, fats, and proteins, the digestive tract is always ready to consume a mixed meal.

Gastric acid is produced when food reaches the stomach. The enzymes pepsin and lipase are released, which aid in the digestion of protein and fat.

Pepsin and lipase are released even if there's no protein or fat in your food, according to study.

The food then enters the small intestine. The stomach's gastric acid is neutralized there, and the intestine is flooded with enzymes that break down proteins, fats, and carbohydrates.

As a result, you don't have to be concerned with your body having to choose between digesting protein and fat or between starches and proteins.
In reality, it's been designed specifically for multitasking.

On Food Changing the Digestive Tract's pH

Another idea behind food pairing is that consuming the wrong foods together can sabotage digestion by creating an acidic environment that prevents certain enzymes from working properly.
Let's start with a refresher on pH. It's a scale that decides whether a solution is acidic or alkaline. The scale ranges from a 0 to 14, with 0 representing the most acidic, 7 indicating neutral, and 14 indicating the most alkaline.
Real, enzymes need a particular pH range to work properly, and not all enzymes in the digestive tract need the same pH range.
Eating foods which are more alkaline or acidic, on the other hand, has no effect on the pH of your digestive tract. The pH of every part of your digestive tract is maintained in a variety of ways by your body.
The stomach, for example, is normally very acidic, with a pH of 1–2.5, but when you consume a meal, it can increase to as high as 5. However, once the pH is brought back down, more gastric acid is easily released.

Maintaining a low pH is important because it aids in the beginning of protein digestion and activates the enzymes released in the stomach. It also aids in the killing of bacteria in your food.

Indeed, the pH within the stomach is so acidic that it is not possible to destroy the stomach lining only with a coating of mucus.

On the other hand, the small intestine is not designed to handle such an acidic environment.

Bicarbonate is applied to the mix until the contents of your intestine hit your small intestine. Bicarbonate is the normal process for your body buffering. It neutralizes gastric acid and retains a pH between 5.5 and 7.8 since it is highly alkaline.

This is the pH that best functions for the enzymes in the small gut.

The body sensors therefore monitor the different acidity levels in the digestive tract.

You can simply make more or more digestive juices in order to achieve the required pH level when you consume the highly acidic or alkaline meal.

On Fermentation of Food in the Stomach

Finally, one of the most common arguments is that incorrect food pairing causes food to ferment or putrefy in the stomach.

When a fast-digesting food is mixed with a slow-digesting food, the fast-digesting food is said to remain in the stomach for so long that it ferments.

This is obviously not the case.

When microorganisms begin to digest your food, fermentation and rotting occur. However, as previously discussed, the stomach has such an acidic pH that the food is effectively sterilized and almost no bacteria can survive.

There is one spot in your digestive tract, however, where bacteria live and fermentation takes place. Trillions of beneficial bacteria reside in your large intestine, also known as your colon.

Some undigested carbohydrates, such as fiber, that were not broken down in your small intestine are fermented by bacteria in your large intestine. As waste, they emit gas and beneficial short-chain fatty acids.

Fermentation is potentially beneficial in this situation. Reduced inflammation, better blood sugar regulation, and a lower risk of colon cancer have all been related to the fatty acids produced by the bacteria.

This also means that the gas you get after eating isn't really a bad thing. It could simply be an indicator that your beneficial bacteria are well fed.

There is no indication that mixing foods has any health benefits. In reality, many of the concepts of modern science are explicitly contradictory.

Examples of Food Combining that Have Been Proven to Work

Although the concepts of food combining diets are not scientifically supported, this does not suggest that the way you mix foods is always insignificant.

For example, there are numerous evidence-based food combinations that can dramatically increase or decrease food digestion and absorption.

Here are a couple of examples

- **Iron and Citrus Fruits**

Heme iron is derived from meat, and non-heme iron, which comes from plant sources, are the two types of iron in the diet.

Heme iron is well absorbed, whereas non-heme iron is poorly absorbed, with absorption rates varying from 1 to 10%. Fortunately, there are many things you could do to boost your iron absorption.

One of the most important things you could do is to supplement with vitamin C.

It functions in two ways. For instance, it promotes the absorption of non-heme iron. Second, it reduces phytic acid's ability to inhibit iron absorption.

This means that mixing vitamin C-rich foods (like citrus fruits or bell peppers) with plant-based iron sources (like spinach, beans, or fortified cereals) is a fantastic idea.

Unfortunately, research has shown that this mixture does not naturally raise iron levels in the body. However, this might simply be as a result that the studies performed so far have been too limited.

- **Carrots and Fats**

Fat is needed for the absorption of certain nutrients, such as fat-soluble vitamins and carotenoids.

Carotenoids are pigments found in fruits and vegetables that are red, orange, or dark green in color. Carrots, onions, red bell peppers, spinach, and broccoli are all good sources.

They've been related to a lower risk of some cancers, heart disease, and vision disorders, among other things.

However, evidence suggests that if you eat these vegetables without any fat — for example, simple carrot sticks or a salad with fat-free dressing — you might be losing out on some of the benefits.

Thc absorption of carotcnoids in fat-frcc, rcduccd-fat, and full-fat dressings was investigated in one study. It was discovered that in order for carotenoids to be absorbed, salad had to be eaten with a fat-containing dressing.

Consume a minimum of five to six grams of fat with carotenoid-containing vegetables to prevent losing out on these essential nutrients.

Toss your salad with some cheese or olive oil, or drizzle a little butter over your steamed broccoli.

- **Dairy Products and Spinach**

Oxalate, an antinutrient that can combine with calcium to form an insoluble compound, is found in foods like spinach, chocolate, and tea.

Depending on the circumstances, this can be beneficial or detrimental to you.

Eating calcium sources such as dairy products and oxalate-containing foods will potentially minimize the risk of developing kidney stones in people who are vulnerable to certain forms of kidney stones.

Combining oxalates and calcium, on the other hand, reduces calcium absorption. In the sense of a well-balanced diet, this is not an issue for most people.

However, this relationship may be troublesome for people who don't consume enough calcium in the first place or who consume a diet rich in oxalates.

Avoid mixing dairy products and other calcium-rich foods with foods high in oxalates if you're worried about getting enough calcium from your diet.

Many food-combination diets aren't founded on scientific evidence. There are, however, a few food combinations that have been clinically proven to influence nutrient digestion and absorption.

The concepts of food pairing are not scientifically proven. The assertion that inappropriate food pairing causes illness and toxins in the body is false.

If you think that the principles of food pairing work well for you, you can keep doing so. There's no need to patch your diet if it's not broken.

Food mixing diets, on the other hand, can be daunting and unmanageable for many people due to the many complicated rules they entail.

Furthermore, there is no proof that they have any distinct advantages.

Food mixing is an eating philosophy of ancient origins that has recently gained a lot of attention.

Proper food combinations, according to proponents of food-combining diets, can lead to illness, toxin accumulation, and digestive distress.

They also agree that the right combinations will help to alleviate these issues.

Is there any validity in these statements, though?

WHAT CAN YOU EAT?

Mealtime for those who consume a regular American diet normally consists of meat and starch. For example, for lunch, a turkey sandwich, or for breakfast, eggs, bacon, and toast. Protein and carbohydrates are seldom consumed together on a food mixing diet.

A food mixing diet recommends eating sweet fruit in moderation and on an empty stomach—a few hours after or 20 minutes before a meal—in addition to keeping proteins and starches apart. Drinking plenty of water is also advised, but not during meals.

What You Should Know

Proponents believe that eating the wrong foods together impairs digestion. As a consequence, undigested food ferments and rots in your stomach. They claim it can cause sickness and/or weight gain, but there is no empirical evidence to back this up.

The rules for mixing foods are rigid and regimented. The fundamental rules must be followed by those who implement these plans. People with dietary conditions, such as celiac disease or gluten sensitivity, will make some changes. As a vegetarian, it could be difficult to adhere to since many plant-based proteins, such as legumes and quinoa, also contain carbohydrates, which is a no-no.

- Meat, fish, poultry, and eggs are all healthy options,non-starchy vegetables ,sour or low-sugar fruit ;
- What to avoid = alcohol , grains and starchy vegetables, such as squash, ,sweet fruit (only in limited amounts) ,refined sugar and processed foods).

Protein

Proteins such as eggs, meat, cheese, and fish can never be eaten with starchy foods such as pasta, rice, squash, or grains.

Grains and starchy vegetables

Just eat cooked non-starchy vegetables like leafy greens with starchy vegetables and other carb-heavy foods like grains and bread (not proteins).

Fruit

Limit the intake of sweet fruits as much as possible. Instead, opt for sour or low-sugar fruits. Nuts, beans, and dried fruit can only be consumed with raw vegetables.

Neutral foods

Dark chocolate, almond milk, egg yolks, cream, coconut water, lemons, butter, and oil are all considered "neutral" foods that can be consumed like any other foods.

Sugar

Restrict the intake of refined sugar and products containing refined sugar. Processed foods, in general, should be avoided because they contain sugars and fats.

Alcohol

Alcohol can be ingested in small quantities. Protein wines, such as dry red and white wines, can only be served with other proteins. Since beer and ale are starchy, they should be paired with other starches or cooked vegetables.

Advantages and disadvantages

Advantages

- Emphasizes whole foods
- Doesn't require carb or calorie counting
- Can help you lose weight

Disadvantages

- Difficult to understand
- Difficult to categorize
- Not viable
- Unsafe for others
- No empirical proof

Food mixing diets, like all restrictive diets, have advantages and disadvantages. Examining the advantages and disadvantages will assist you in making an educated decision about whether or not to try this eating plan.

The focus is on whole foods, which is a plus

Following this diet would almost certainly result in a higher intake of whole foods. The protocol forbids the intake of all foods containing added sugars, which excludes a significant number of processed foods.

When food is consumed closer to its natural state, it is often easier to keep different forms of food apart from one another. Protein, carbohydrates, and various forms of fat are typically contained in processed foods.

There are no carbs or calories to count

There's no point counting calories or carbohydrates, and portion control isn't required, making this otherwise complicated eating plan much easier to follow.

Might Help You Lose Weight

A strict set of guidelines may aid in making more mindful food choices. It is possible to eat less calories and lose weight by removing empty calories and carefully preparing meals and snacks. However, it's possible that this has nothing to do with food pairing. Any weight loss you experience on this plan is more likely due to a calorie deficit (consuming less calories than you burn) rather than specific food combinations.

It's Hard to Adopt

The diet's guidelines are confusing and may be difficult to obey for certain people. This diet is difficult to follow because of its impracticality, as well as the need to give up some comfort foods and remember when it's OK to drink water and when it's OK to eat fruit.

Categorization Is Difficult

The majority of foods aren't simply acidic or alkaline. Spinach, for example, is alkaline while also providing protein to the body (most proteins are considered acidic). Quinoa is a grain that contains both starchy carbohydrates and protein. It's almost impossible to neatly categorize foods using this plan's guidelines.

Not a long-term solution

These kinds of diets are incredibly difficult to adhere to. As a consequence, keeping to a food mixing diet for the long term can be challenging. Furthermore, any weight loss achieved when following this restrictive diet is likely to reappear once normal eating habits are restored.

Some People Find It Dangerous

Food combinations should be avoided by people with such medical conditions. People with diabetes shouldn't only eat carbs; they also need protein or fat to prevent their blood sugar levels from rising too high. Before attempting this diet, consult your doctor if you have a chronic health problem.

There is no scientific evidence

Proteins and carbohydrates are digested at different speeds, according to proponents of food mixing, making it harder for the body to absorb them when eaten together. They also say that different foods respond differently to different pH levels in the intestine. As a result, combining two foods that require different pH levels won't allow them to be digested together. Obviously, none of these convictions were supported by empirical evidence.

The digestive system (which includes saliva in the mouth, stomach acids, small intestine enzymes, and large intestine bacteria) works together to absorb food and make it available for the rest of the body. It is capable of completing this task without the need for food mixing.

CHAPTER 7

~CONSUMING WATER REGULARLY BUT ALSO TEAS BENEFICIAL TO THE BODY~

It is important to remain hydrated for good health and well-being, but many people do not drink enough fluids on a regular basis.

Water makes up about 60% of the human body, and it covers about 71 percent of the planet's surface.

It's possible that the abundant existence of water means that getting enough water per day isn't at the first on many people's priority lists.

Facts about water consumption

- ✓ We are 60 percent water as adults, and our blood is 90 percent water;
- ✓ Water is important for the kidneys and other bodily functions;
- ✓ When the skin is dehydrated, it's more susceptible to skin conditions and wrinkling;

- ✓ Drinking water instead of soda would help with weight loss.

Drinking water has a lot of advantages

Drinking water has a variety of health benefits, including kidney health and weight loss.All of the body's cells and organs need water to function properly.

Here's why our bodies need water:

1. It keeps the joints lubricated

Cartilage, which is present in joints and spinal disks, contains around 80% water. Long-term dehydration can reduce the ability of the joints to absorb shock, resulting in joint pain.

2. It is responsible for the production of saliva and mucus

Saliva assists in food digestion and keeps the mouth, nose, and eyes moist. Friction and damage are avoided as a result. Water also helps to keep the mouth clean. It could also help to prevent tooth decay when consumed instead of sweetened drinks.

3.It also transports oxygen in the body

Blood is more than 90% water, and it transports oxygen to all areas of the body.

4. It improves the protection and appearance of the skin

The skin may become more susceptible to skin disorders and premature wrinkling as a result of dehydration.

5. It protects the brain, spinal cord, and other delicate tissues by cushioning them

Dehydration may have an effect on the structure and function of the brain. It's also involved in hormone and neurotransmitter development. Dehydration for an extended period of time may cause issues with reasoning and thinking.

6. It keeps the body's temperature in control

When the body heats up, water contained in the middle layers of the skin rises to the surface as sweat. It cools the body as it evaporates. In sports, for example.

Some scientists believe that when the body has too little water, heat storage increases and the individual's ability to withstand heat stress decreases.

If heat stress occurs during exercise, a large amount of water in the body can help to reduce physical strain. However, further research into these effects is needed.

7. It is necessary for the digestive system to work properly

Water is needed for proper bowel function. Dehydration can cause digestive issues, constipation, and a stomach that is too acidic. Heartburn and stomach ulcers are more likely as a result of this.

8. It removes waste from the body

Sweating, as well as the removal of urine and feces, require water.

9. It aids in the maintenance of blood pressure

Water deficiency can cause blood to thicken, raising blood pressure.

10. It is required by the airways

When you're dehydrated, your body restricts your airways to prevent water loss. Asthma and allergies can become worse as a result of this.

11. It facilitates the intake of minerals and nutrients

These dissolve in water, allowing them to enter various parts of the body.

12. It protects the kidneys from damage

The kidneys are in charge of regulating fluid in the body. Kidney stones and other problems may result from a lack of water.

13. It improves athletic results

Some scientists believe that drinking more water will help you perform better during strenuous exercise.

While further research is required to confirm this, one study found that dehydration decreases efficiency in activities lasting more than 30 minutes.

14. Loss of weight

If you drink water instead of sweetened juices and sodas, you might lose weight. By generating a feeling of fullness, "preloading" with water before meals will help avoid overeating.

15. It lessens the risk of a hangover

When partying, unsweetened sparkling water with ice and lemon can be substituted for alcoholic beverages to help stop alcohol overconsumption.

Harm to the kidneys

Water aids in the dissolution of minerals and nutrients, allowing them to be more readily absorbed by the body. It also assists in removing waste materials.

The kidneys works for the maintenance of fluid balance.

Water is important for the kidneys because of these two roles.

The kidneys filter between 120-150 quarts of fluid every day.

The body excretes about 1-2 quarts in the form of urine, while the remainder is recovered via the bloodstream.

The kidneys need water to function properly.

Waste products and excess fluid would build up within the body if the kidneys do not function properly.

Chronic kidney disease, if left untreated, can lead to kidney failure. When the kidneys stop functioning, dialysis or a kidney transplant are needed.

Urinary tract infections (UTIs) are the body's second most widespread infection. Per year, they account for nearly 8.1 million visits to health-care facilities in the United States.

Permanent damage can occur if infections spread to the upper urinary tract, including the kidneys. Kidney infections that occur suddenly or acutely can be fatal, particularly if septicemia develops.

An easy way to lower the risk of developing a UTI and to help treat an existing UTI is to drink plenty of water.

Kidney stones obstruct the kidneys' ability to function properly. When present, it can make UTIs more difficult to treat.

These more complex UTIs usually necessitate a longer course of antibiotics, ranging from 7 to 14 days.

A lack of water is the most common cause of kidney stones. The majority of people who mention them do not drink the recommended amount of water per day. Chronic kidney disease can be exacerbated by kidney stones.

The American College of Physicians released new recommendations in November 2014 for people who have previously developed kidney stones. According to the recommendations, raising fluid intake to allow for 2 liters of urination per day could reduce the risk of stone recurrence in half with no side effects.

Dehydration occurs when we use and lose more water than our bodies can absorb. It can create an electrolyte imbalance in the body. Potassium, phosphate, and sodium are electrolytes that assist in the transmission of electrical signals between cells. When the kidneys work properly, they keep the body's electrolyte levels in check.

These electrical signals become jumbled when the kidneys are unable to maintain a balance of electrolyte levels. Seizures, including involuntary muscle movements and loss of consciousness, can result.

Dehydration can lead to renal failure, which can be fatal in severe cases. Anemia, central nervous system injuries, heart failure, and compromised immune systems are all possible complications of chronic kidney failure.

~SOURCES~

Some of the water needed by the body is obtained from high-water-content foods like soups, tomatoes, and oranges, but the majority is obtained from drinking water and other beverages.

Water is lost by the body during normal functioning, and it must be replaced. We lose water from things like sweating and urination, but we also lose water when we breathe.

The best fluid source for the body is water, whether it comes from the tap or a bottle.

Milk and juices are also healthy sources of fluid, but alcoholic and caffeine-containing beverages, such as soft drinks, coffee, and beer, are not recommended because they often contain empty calories. Weight loss can be aided by drinking water instead of soda.

Caffeinated drinks were historically believed to have diuretic properties, meaning they caused the body to release water. Caffeinated beverages, on the other hand, have been shown to cause limited fluid loss in studies.

The quantity of water required each day varies depending on how active a person is, how much they sweat, and other factors.

As there is no set amount of water which must be ingested each day, there is widespread consensus about what constitutes a balanced fluid intake.

Reasons Why You Should Drink More Tea, According To Science

Tea is more than just a familiar hot beverage in the winter. Tea has been a practice and custom in cultures all over the world for thousands of years, and it still is today.
Tea was first eaten in China, perhaps as early as 2737 B.C., and then spread to Japan, Holland, and finally the rest of Europe. Tea was first brought to America by Dutch settlers in 1650. While tea was heavily taxed at first, Britain was one of the last European countries to introduce it. The majority of tea imports were illegally imported until the British government lowered the tax rate in 1784, allowing tea to become a drink for all rather than only the rich.

Every day, approximately 75 million cups of tea are drunk in the United Kingdom, with over 3 billion cups consumed worldwide. Tea's success is due to more than just its good flavor. It has been consumed for centuries because of its medicinal properties, which have now been extensively researched. So, let's go over all the scientific explanations why you should drink more tea.

There are various health benefits of drinking tea

Tea seems to be able to solve just about any problem. Have you had a particularly trying day at work? Curl up with a hot beverage. Do you have a sluggish feeling? A matcha latte will perk you up. Are you feeling under the weather? Tea and honey will help to soothe a sore throat.

Tea's medicinal properties, regardless of variety, have been recognized for thousands of years. Many of those advantages are now backed up by modern research.

Here are ten scientifically validated reasons to increase your tea consumption √

1. It increases the metabolic rate

Polyphenols found in black, oolong, and green tea have all been shown to increase calorie intake and minimize body fat. Tea, it turns out, encourages one kind of fat in particular: brown fat. Brown fat is more metabolically active and contains more mitochondria than white fat, so it can help you lose calories and increase your metabolism.

According to a study of 15 reports, those who drank two to six cups of green tea per day for more than 12 weeks had lower body fat and weight than those who did not. Still not a fan of brewed tea? Green tea extract, a conc. form of green tea found in powders and tablets has also been shown to help people lose weight by increasing their metabolism.

2. It has anti-inflammatory properties

Anything from diabetes to cognitive impairment has been related to inflammation. It has also been linked to the cause of nearly all chronic diseases. Tea's antioxidant polyphenols are effective anti-inflammatory agents. In fact, the antioxidant strength of EGCG in green tea is up to 100 times greater than that of vitamin C.

Tea has been shown to assist people with inflammatory bowel disease and other inflammation-related diseases.

3. It lowers the risk of dying from such chronic diseases

Regular tea intake was found to lower the risk of death from heart disease, stroke, and some cancers in a study of over 40,000 adults. Participants who drank five or more cups of green tea a day had a 16 percent lower risk of mortality due to cardiovascular disorders than those who drank less than one cup per day, according to the report. Green tea's protective role is attributed to its effect on hypertension and obesity, as well as its strong polyphenols.

Chronic diseases are part of the main causes of death in the United States, making it even more important to drink tea on a regular basis. Those who drank three to four cups a day had more benefits than those who drank one cup or none at all, so drink up!

4. It has the potential to enhance insulin sensitivity

Green tea can aid in the reduction of diabetes complications. Diabetes is a global health crisis that can lead to severe complications, early death, and a lower quality of life. Tea has been shown to highten insulin sensitivity, protect pancreatic cells from more damage, and minimize inflammation, all of which are helpful to people who are at risk of or have diabetes.

5. It is beneficial to your mental health

Tea consumption on a regular basis may reduce the risk of Alzheimer's disease and other neurodegenerative diseases. Although the real causes of Alzheimer's disease are unknown and there is no cure, studies show that drinking green and black tea increases cognitive scores in people with dementia and Alzheimer's disease.

It may also help to reduce cognitive loss by improving memory and attention span. Tea has been shown to enhance reaction time, visual processing, memory, and concentration when caffeine and L-theanine are combined. It also changes the brain structure to allow for more effective data processing.

6. It can aid in the prevention of cancer

The catechin EGCG in green tea is a strong antioxidant with cancer-fighting properties. EGCG has been shown in lab and animal studies to minimize metastasis and improve outcomes in cancers of the breasts, lungs, colon, skin, and other organs.

While further human clinical trials are required, several long-term observational studies have discovered similar cancer-fighting benefits. For example, Japanese women who consumed ten or more cups of green tea per day had a seven-year delay in the onset of cancer. This amount of tea is equal to 2.5 grams of green tea extract, according to sources.

7. It is beneficial to your oral health

Sugary sodas and juices, for example, are not all good for your mouth. Teas, on the other hand, can help with oral health. Fluoride in tea can help to boost bacterial communities in the mouth. Periodontal disorder, cavities, and likely oral cancer are all minimized as a result of this. If you drink tea, you can feel good about your oral health even if you don't floss every now and then.

8. It has the potential to increase fertility

Is there something that tea can't accomplish? According to a 2018 study, the degree of oxidative stress in reproductive tissues has a major effect on fertility issues. Then there's tea. Tea polyphenols have been shown to have anti-inflammatory and antioxidant properties. As a result, the authors believe that tea will help both men and women become more fertile. More research is required, but it appears to be encouraging.

9. It hydrates the body

This one could catch you off guard. Though it was once believed that tea (and coffee) contributed to dehydration by serving as a diuretic and making the body to lose more fluid, new research shows that drinking six to eight cups of tea per day is just as hydrating as drinking the same amount of water.

10. It's helpful to the digestive system

Fiber and probiotics aren't the only things that can help your gut. Tea polyphenols have been shown in experiments to change gut bacteria for the better.

Reduced carbohydrate absorption, increased blood sugar levels, and weight loss are all potential health benefits.

What are the various kinds of tea?

What kind of tea should you have now that you're craving a warm mug of tea? Black, green, oolong, and white teas are the four primary types of tea (excluding herbal teas, which could be produced from a large variety of plants).

The leaves of the evergreen shrub *Camellia sinensis* are used in all four forms, although they are processed differently.

1. **White tea**

This is the least processed tea type made from the Camellia sinensis plant, and it has a milder taste and less caffeine than black tea (though caffeine levels vary among brands). The leaves for white tea are picked while still coated in silvery-white hairs.

2. **Green tea**

The polyphenols, a class of phytochemicals having strong antioxidant properties, are preserved when fresh green tea leaves are steamed. Flavonoids make up the rest of the polyphenols in green tea. Catechins are the kind of flavonoids that have the most heart health benefits, and green tea has a lot of them! The most well-known and researched catechin is epigallocatechin gallate (EGCG). Green tea, like white tea, contains a small amount of caffeine, varying from 25 to 35 mg per cup.
Matcha is basically green tea powder, but unlike brewed green tea, the tea leaves are covered prior to harvest, resulting in a more concentrated taste and higher caffeine and antioxidant levels.

3. ***Oolong tea***

Oolong tea is made from partly fermented tea leaves and has a caffeine content equivalent to white and green tea. Though less well-known, oolong tea has many of the same health benefits as the more well-studied green tea.

4. **Black tea**

This is the most processed of the tea leaves, the polyphenols in it provide unique benefits. All teas derived the *Camellia sinensis* plant contain more caffeine than black tea.

Black tea's caffeine content, combined with its processing, has shown to be more effective than other teas in preventing and treating obesity.

Side effects and safety

While most people are healthy drinking up to six cups of tea a day, some herbal teas contain plants that can cause allergic reactions in some people.
Those allergic to the daisy family or ragweed, for example, should avoid dandelion tea.

Some problems to remember are:

1.Caffeine is a stimulant

Caffeine content varies by tea and brand, but black tea has the most. White, gray, and oolong teas have the lowest levels of caffeine, with just 25 to 35 mg per 8-ounce cup. Caffeine allergy or sensitivity sufferers should stick to herbal, white, green, or oolong teas in the afternoon and evening and avoid caffeinated teas.

2.Deficiency in iron

Anemia is a condition of which there is a lack. Tea (and coffee) contain tannins and caffeine, which can reduce iron absorption, particularly from plant sources. Tea consumption should be avoided by vegetarians, vegans, and those suffering from anemia.

Children, to be precise. Although the FDA does not have any recommendations for healthy caffeine consumption for children, the European Food Information Council states that, depending on age, children should drink one to two cups of tea a day without exceeding safe caffeine limits.

3.Heat damage

Have you heard about the connection between hot beverages and cancer risk in the news?

According to a 2016 report, anyone who drank tea less than four minutes after pouring or at temperatures above 65 degrees Celsius had a higher risk of esophageal cancer (150 degrees Fahrenheit). Despite this and other studies, sips of beverages below 150 degrees Fahrenheit (65 degrees Celsius), which can be obtained by waiting five or more minutes after steeping period until ingestion, tend to be secure.

Regardless of the tea you choose, the analysis is conclusive. To stay warm in the winter, cool off in the summer, and enjoy a healthy heart, brain, and body, drink three to six cups of white, green, oolong, black, or herbal tea every day.

PART III

~THE WEIGHT LOSS-FOOD PLAN TO FOLLOW~

If you're trying to lose weight, meal preparation can be useful. When done correctly, it will help you reach the requisite calorie deficit for weight loss while supplying your body the necessary nutrients it needs to work and stay healthy.

Meal planning ahead of time will help you save time and ease the meal preparation process.

How to Make a Weight Loss Meal Plan

The sheer number of choices available when it comes to weight loss meal plans can be daunting. When looking for the best strategy, there are a few things to bear in mind.

Creating a calorie deficit that is both nutrient-dense and calorie-dense

All weight-loss programs have one thing in common: they encourage you to consume less calories than you expend.

However, while a calorie deficit can aid weight loss regardless of how it is achieved, what you consume is as important how much you eat. That's because the foods you eat play a big role in meeting your nutrient requirements.

Any universal guidelines should be followed by a successful weight loss meal plan:

• Contains a lot of protein and fiber. Foods high in protein and fiber make you stay fuller for longer, reducing cravings and encouraging you to consume smaller portions.
• Avoids processed foods and sugary drinks. These foods have high calories but low nutrients, so they don't stimulate your brain's fullness centers, making it difficult to lose weight or meet your nutrient needs.
• Contains a wide range of fruits and vegetables. Both have high water and fiber, which help you feel satisfied. These nutrient-dense foods often make meeting your daily nutrient needs a lot easier.

Creating nutrient-dense dishes

Start by filling 1/3 to 1/2 of your plate with non-starchy vegetables to instill these tips into your meal plan. They have calories and have plenty of water, fiber and vitamins and minerals.

Fill your plate to 1/4 to 1/3 with protein-rich foods such as beef, fish, tofu, seitan or legumes, and the rest with whole grains, berries or starchy vegetables. These include additional proteins, vitamins, minerals and fiber.

A splash of healthy fats from foods like avocados, olives, nuts, and seeds will enhance the flavor of your meal.

Some people can benefit from a snack to help them get through the time between meals. Snacks high in protein and fiber seem to be the most powerful for weight loss.

Apple slices of peanut butter, vegetables and hummus, roasted chickpeas or Greek yogurt with fruit and nuts are all good options.

Meal preparation tips that will help meal planning work for you

The ability of a good weight loss meal plan to help you hold the weight off is critical.

Here are several ideas for increasing the long-term feasibility of your meal plan.

Choose a meal-planning approach that works for you

Meal preparation can be accomplished in a number of ways, so choose the one that best suits your schedule.

You may want to batch cook all of your meals over the weekend so that you can catch individual portions during the week. Alternatively, if you choose to cook every day, prepping all of your ingredients ahead of time might be the best option for you.

If you don't like following recipes and want a little more versatility, consider a strategy that lets you stock your refrigerator and pantry with unique portions of foods each week while allowing you to improvise when putting meals together.

Grocery shopping in bulk is another time-saving tactic that keeps your refrigerator and pantry stocked with nutrient-dense foods.

Consider downloading an app

Apps could be a reasonable addition to your meal-planning toolkit. Meal plan templates are included in some applications, which you can customize based on your food preferences or allergies. They could also be a useful tool for keeping track of your favorite recipes and storing all of your details in one place.

Furthermore, several apps generate personalized shopping lists based on your favorite recipes or what's left in your fridge, saving you time and reducing food waste.

Choose an appropriate number of recipes

Choosing a sufficient number of recipes means that you have ample variety without spending any of your spare time in the kitchen.

Look at your calendar to see how many days you're likely to eat out — whether for a date, a client dinner, or brunch with friends — while determining how many meals to plan.

Divide the remaining breakfasts, lunches, and dinners by the amount of meals you will cook or plan realistically for the week. This would help you figure out how many portions of each meal you'll need to prepare.

Then, to choose your recipes, simply sift through your cookbooks or online food blogs.

Think of treats

Allowing yourself to become excessively hungry in between meals can lead to overeating at your next meal, making weight loss more difficult.

Snacks will help you consume less calories a day by reducing hunger, increasing feelings of fullness, and lowering your total calorie intake.

Combinations high in protein and fiber, such as almonds, roasted chickpeas, or vegetables and hummus, prove to be the best for weight loss.

Bear in mind, though, that some people gain weight when they add snacks to their diet. As a result, keep watch of your performance while using this technique.

Ensure that there is a wide range of options

Eating a diverse diet is important for supplying the body with the nutrients it needs.

As a result, meal plans that prescribe batch cooking 1–2 recipes for the whole week should be avoided. This lack of variety could make it difficult to meet your daily nutrient needs and, over time, boredom, reducing the sustainability of your meal plan.

Instead, make sure your daily meal contains a range of foods.

Reduce the time you spend preparing meals

Meal preparation does not have to entail spending a lot of time in the kitchen. Here are a few ideas for cutting down on meal prep time.

Maintain a consistent schedule. Setting aside specific times to prepare the week's meals, go grocery shopping, and cook will help you make better choices and streamline your meal planning.

- ✓ Make a grocery list before going shopping. Grocery lists that are detailed will help you save time while shopping. To avoid returning to a previously visited section, arrange your list by supermarket divisions.
- ✓ Choose recipes that are compatible. When batch cooking, choose recipes that call for a variety of appliances. For example, one recipe might call for the oven, no more than two stovetop burners, and no heating at all.
- ✓ Make a schedule for when you'll be cooking. Organize your workflow by beginning with the recipe that takes the most cooking time and working your way down. Cooking times can be cut even further with electric pressure cookers or slow cookers.
- ✓ Recipes that could be prepared in 15–20 minutes from start to finish are ideal for inexperienced cooks or those who just want to spend less time in the kitchen.

Safely store and reheat your meals

Safely preserving and reheating your meals will help preserve their taste while also lowering your risk of food poisoning.

To bear in mind, here are some government-approved food safety guidelines:

- ✓ Make sure the food is properly cooked. Most meats should be cooked to a temperature of at least 165°F (75°C) to kill the majority of bacteria.
- ✓ Place frozen food inside the refrigerator to thaw. Bacteria can multiply when frozen foods or meals are thawed on the counter. If you're low of time, submerge foods in cold water for 30 minutes, then change the water.
- ✓ Reheat food in a healthy manner. Before feeding, make sure your meals are reheated to at least 165°F (75°C). Defrosted frozen meals should be consumed within 24 hours.
- ✓ Get rid of stale food. Refrigerated meals should be eaten in 3–4 days of cooking, and frozen meals within 3–6 months of freezing.

Recipes that are easy to prepare

Recipes for weight loss don't have to be difficult. Here are a few easy-to-make recipes that only require a few ingredients.

Soups are a great choice. Soups could be prepared in bulk and frozen in individual servings. Include a range of fruits, as well as beef, fish, beans, peas, and lentils. If desired, serve with brown rice, quinoa, or potatoes.

- ✓ Pizza made from scratch. Start with a veggie or whole-grain crust, a thin layer of sauce, a protein source like tempeh or turkey breast, and vegetables. Serve with new leafy greens and a little cheese on top.
- ✓ Salads are delicious. Salads are convenient and adaptable. Begin with leafy greens, colorful vegetables, and a protein source. Attach nuts, beans, whole grains, or starchy vegetables to the top with olive oil and vinegar.
- ✓ Pasta is a tasty dish. Start with your favorite whole-grain pasta and a protein source like chicken, fish, or tofu. Then add some vegetables like broccoli or spinach, as well as a tomato-based pasta sauce or pesto.
- ✓ Recipes for using a slow cooker or an electric pressure cooker. Chili, enchiladas, spaghetti sauce, and stew can all be made with these. Simply put your ingredients in your system, turn it on, and let it take care of the rest.
- ✓ Bowls for grains. Cook grains like quinoa or brown rice in bulk, then top with non-starchy vegetables, chicken, or hard-boiled eggs, and a nutritious dressing of your choosing.

The recipes mentioned above are easy to prepare and take very little time. They're also highly flexible because they can be prepared in a number of ways.

Dietary constraints suggestions

Plant-based substitutes such as tofu, tempeh, seitan, beans, flax or chia seeds, as well as vegetable-based milk and yogurt can usually replace beef, fish, eggs and dairy products.

Quinoa, millet, oats, buckwheat, amaranth, teff, corn and sorghum can be utilized rather than gluten-containing grains and flours.

Lower-carb grains and starchy vegetables can be substituted for carb-rich grains and vegetables.

Try replacing pasta with spiralized noodles or spaghetti squash, cauliflower rice with couscous or rice, lettuce leaves with taco shells, and seaweed or rice paper with tortilla wraps.

Bear in mind that eliminating a food group entirely can necessitate supplementation to meet your daily nutrient requirements.

Nutrient-dense, protein- and fiber-rich weight-loss meals should be consumed. This meal plan can be modified to fit a variety of dietary restrictions, but fully eliminating a food category will necessitate supplementation.

A healthy weight loss meal plan keeps you in a calorie deficit while also supplying all of the nutrients you need.

When done correctly, it can be extremely easy and time-saving.

Choosing a weight-loss approach that works for you will also help you avoid regaining weight.

Overall, meal preparation is an extremely effective weight-loss technique.

~WEIGHT LOSS FOOD RECIPES~

1.Instant Pot Shrimp and Broccoli

Ingredients

- 1 pound fresh or frozen shrimp
- 2 crowns of broccoli
- 1/4 cup of soy sauce
- 2 minced garlic cloves
- 2 tbsp. grated fresh ginger
- Oyster sauce, 2 tbsp.
- Brown sugar, 2 tsp.
- Rice wine vinegar, 1 tsp
- Seeds of sesame
- Sriracha sauce
- Onion green

Instructions

1. Separate the broccoli crowns into florets.

2.If you purchased fresh shrimp, lean your hands before deshelling them. If you bought it frozen, be sure to let it thaw in the refrigerator overnight. If they need to be deshelled, go ahead and do that as well.

3. Combine the soy sauce, minced garlic, ginger, oyster sauce, brown sugar, and rice wine vinegar in your Instant Pot. To mix the ingredients, whisk them together.
4. In the Instant Pot, add the broccoli and shrimp. Seal the Instant Pot and cook for 1 minute on high pressure (Manual or Pressure Cook).
5. When the buzzer sounds, automatically release the pressure.
6. To keep it low-carb, serve the shrimp and broccoli with rice or cauliflower rice, sriracha, sesame seeds, and sliced green onion.

2.Protein Pancakes

Ingredients

- 1 egg
- 1 rounded scoop of protein powder
- A half-cup of oats
- 1/4 cup greek yogurt, simple
- 1/3 gallon of milk
- 1 tblsp baking soda
- 1 teaspoon of cinnamon
- 1 tsp vanilla extract (optional)

Instructions

1. In a high-powered blender, mix all of the ingredients.

2. Preheat a griddle to medium-high heat. Using a flat pan on the stove instead of a griddle if you don't have one. Cooking spray or melted butter may be used to coat the hot griddle (or pan).

3. Pour 1/4 cup of the batter onto the griddle for perfect-sized pancakes.

4. Flip the pancakes as the tops of the pancakes begin to bubble.

3.Sautéed Mushrooms Grilled Cheese

Ingredients

- 12 tbsp extra virgin olive oil
- 2 cups sliced cremini mushrooms
- Salt and black pepper to taste.
- 8 rye bread slices
- 2 cups Swiss cheese, shredded
- 1 cup of onions, caramelized
- 12 tbsp thyme leaves, new (optional)
- 2 tbsp butter (softened)

Instructions

1. Inside a skillet, heat up the olive oil over medium heat.

2. Cook for about 6 minutes, or until the mushrooms are beautifully caramelized. Salt and pepper to taste.

3. On a cutting board, lay out four slices of rye bread.

4. Place half of the Swiss on top, followed by the onions and mushrooms. Add the remaining cheese and the thyme (if using).

5. Finish with the remaining rye slices.

6. Butter all sides of the sandwiches with softened butter.
7. Preheat a medium-low heat in a large cast-iron or nonstick skillet.
8. Cook the sandwiches for 5 to 6 minutes per hand, working in batches if necessary, until thoroughly toasted and golden brown.

4.Breakfast Veggie Burger

Ingredients

- 1 veggie burger patty
- 1 thick tomato slice
- 3 thin red onion slices
- A quarter avocado, sliced
- 1 tablespoon canola oil
- 1big egg
- black pepper, freshly roasted

Instructions

1. In a cast-iron skillet, heat the oil over medium heat. Cook the patty for a period of three minutes on each hand, or until browned. Serve the tomato slice on a plate with sliced onion and the veggie patty on top.
2. Inside a nonstick skillet, heat up the oil over medium-low heat. Crack the egg softly into the skillet. Cook on low heat for a period of three to five minutes, or until the white is fully set.

3. Place the egg atop the burger. Add the parsley and black pepper to taste. Serve with a side of avocado.

5.Chicken Potstickers

Ingredients

- 24 pot stickers (frozen) (chicken, pork, or vegetable)
- 1 tbsp peanut or sesame oil
- 4 oz (preferably shiitake) mushrooms, stems cut, sliced
- 2 cups of sugar snap or snow peas, trimmed of rough ends
- 1 tablespoon of soy sauce
- 1 tbsp vinegar de vinaigre de riz (rice wine vinegar)
- sriracha to taste
- seeds of sesame (optional) (Sesame seeds are rich in magnesium, which helps to relieve stress and lower blood pressure.)
- scallions, cut (optional)

Instructions

1. Fill a large saucepan halfway through with water and bring to a boil. Cook for a few minutes, until the pot stickers are tender but not gummy. Drain the water.
2. In a large nonstick skillet or sauté pan, heat the oil over medium heat.
3. Cook for 2 to 3 minutes, until the mushrooms are lightly browned.

4. Add the cooked potstickers to the pan and cook, stirring occasionally, until the bottoms are crispy and golden, around 2 to 3 minutes per hand.
5. Throw in the snap peas and heat up in the last minute of cooking.
6. Stir in the soy sauce, vinegar, and sriracha after removing the pan from the oven.
7. Divide amongst four bowls and then top with sesame seeds and scallions (if using).

6.Swedish Turkey Meatballs

Ingredients

- 2 white bread slices, cut into small pieces
- 12 cup Milk with 2% fat
- 12 ounces of field chuck
- 12 oz turkey ground
- 1 minced small onion
- 2 garlic cloves, minced
- 12 tsp nutmeg powder
- 1 teaspoon of salt
- A quarter teaspoon of black pepper
- 1 tablespoon of butter
- 2 tablespoons flour
- 12 cup beef stock (low sodium)
- 1 tbsp yogurt (Greek)

- for serving, use cranberry or raspberry marmalade (optional)

Instructions

1. In a tub, combine the bread and 14 cup milk and soak for 5 minutes.
2. Drain and squeeze out some of the moisture consumed by the bread with your hands (it should be moist, not sopping).
3. Combine the bread, beef, turkey, onion, garlic, nutmeg, salt, and pepper in a mixing bowl.
4. Kindly combine all ingredients, then roll into golf ball-sized meatballs.
5. In a large nonstick sauté pan or skillet, melt the butter over medium heat.
6. Add the meatballs and cook for about 10 minutes, turning periodically, until well browned on all sides and cooked through.
7. Put the meatballs on a plate and set aside.
8. Mix in the flour with a whisk or a wooden spoon until it is uniformly distributed in the remaining fat throughout the pan.
9. Slowly pour in the stock, stirring regularly to avoid lumps.
10. Stir in the remaining 14 cup milk and cook for 3 minutes, or until the flour thickens the liquid.
11. Stir in the yogurt, then return the meatballs to the pan and cook for another 10 minutes, or until the sauce is sticking to the meatballs tightly.

12. Serve with boiled potatoes or lightly buttered noodles, or on their own. If using, pass the marmalade around the table.

7.Grilled Chicken Avocado Salad

Ingredients

- fried chicken, 12 oz
- 12 c. arugula (arugula) (1 prewashed bag)
- 14 cup cranberries, dried
- 1 pitted, peeled, and sliced avocado
- 14 cup goat cheese, crumbled
- 14 cup coarsely chopped walnuts
- 14 cup vinaigrette with honey and mustard
- Salt and black pepper to taste.

Instructions

Inside a large mixing bowl, combine the chicken, arugula, cranberries, avocado, goat cheese, walnuts, vinaigrette, salt, and pepper, and thoroughly add the dressing with your hands or 2 forks.

8.Chicken Vegetables Pasta with Alfredo Sauce

Ingredients

- 2 tbsp butter (unsalted)
- 3 tablespoons flour

- 3 mugs Milk with 2% fat
- 2 garlic cloves, chopped
- 2 tbsp Parmesan cheese, grated
- salt and black pepper to taste.
- 12 tbsp extra virgin olive oil
- 2 cups broccoli florets, sliced into bite-size pieces
- 8 oz. sliced cremini mushrooms
- 14 cup sun-dried tomatoes, chopped
- 8 oz. thinly sliced cooked chicken breast (store-bought rotisserie chicken works well)
- whole-wheat fettuccine (12 oz)

Instructions

1. Melt the butter inside a saucepan over medium-low heat to make the béchamel.
2. Add the flour and whisk to mix. One minute of cooking, slowly whisk in the milk to avoid any lumps. Stir in the garlic and cook, whisking often, for 10 to 15 minutes, or until the sauce has thickened nicely.
3. Season using salt and pepper and stir the Parmesan in. Keep yourself wet.
4. In a large skillet or sauté pan, heat the oil over medium-high heat.
5. Cook for 3 to 4 minutes after adding the broccoli. Toss in the tomatoes and mushrooms.

6. Continue to cook for another 5 minutes, or until the vegetables are lightly caramelized.
7. Add the chicken and mix well. Salt and pepper to taste.
8. In the meantime, prepare the pasta according to the package directions.
9. Drain and set aside 1 cup of the cooking liquid.

Return the pasta to the pot and then toss with the sauce and chicken mixture to coat.

10. If the sauce is too thick, thin it with some of the pasta water. Serve right away.

9.Spicy-Sweet Grilled Chicken and Pineapple Sandwich

Ingredients

- 4 chicken breasts, boneless and skinless (4–6 oz each)
- Sauce teriyaki
- 4 Swiss cheese slices
- 4 12" thick pineapple slices
- 4 buns (whole-wheat) (Note: Whole-wheat buns are often made with a low percentage of whole grains and a large amount of sugar.) Choose a brand with 3 grams of fiber per bun and less than 110 calories.
- 1 thinly sliced red onion

Instructions

1. Inside a resealable plastic bag, mix the chicken and enough teriyaki sauce to cover, and marinate for a minimum of thirty minutes and up to 12 hours.
2. Preheat the grill until it's very hot (you shouldn't be able to keep your hand above the grates for above five seconds.)
3. Put the chicken on the grill after removing it from the marinade; remove any remaining marinade.
4. Cook for 4 to 5 minutes on the first side, then flip and add the cheese to each breast immediately.
5. Cook until the cheese has melted and the chicken is lightly charred and firm to the touch, around 5 minutes. Remove the item and set it aside.
6. Add the pineapple and buns to the grill while the chicken rests. Cook for around 2 minutes per hand, until the buns are lightly toasted and the pineapple is soft and caramelized.
7. Place chicken, red onion, jalapeo slices, and pineapple slices on top of each bun. Drizzle the chicken with a little more teriyaki sauce if desired.

10.Instant Pot Steak Fajitas

Ingredients

- 1 tablespoon extra virgin olive oil
- 1 thinly sliced flank steak

- 1 onion, sliced
- 1 red pepper, sliced
- 1 green pepper, sliced
- taco seasoning (1 tbsp)
- 1/2 gallon beef stock
- 1 tablespoon of tomato paste
- to eat, tortillas and lime wedges

Instructions

1. Turn on the Instant Pot's Saute feature. Add the olive oil after it has warmed up.
2. Cook the steak in the Instant Pot for no more than 2 minutes. It's fine if the steak isn't fully cooked.
3. Add the beef broth and the tomato paste to the pot. Mix until all of the tomato paste is mixed into the broth.
4. Toss in the sliced red, green, and onion, as well as the taco seasoning.
5. Cover the Instant Pot using the lid and set it to seal. Cook the steak for 10 minutes at high pressure on manual (Pressure Cook). When the Instant Pot reaches pressure, it will cook for the amount of time you choose.
6. When the timer beeps, immediately release the pressure.
7. Serve with tortillas or in a bowl with a bed of greens and guacamole if you want to keep it low-carb.

PART IV

~ACTIVE LIFESTYLE: PHYSICAL EXERCISE AND GETTING MOVING~

If you spend your days hobbling in agony from your bed to your reclining chair and back, vigorous exercise can be the last thing on your mind. Being involved, on the other hand, can dramatically improve your fitness, comfort, mobility, and overall quality of life. Here are five activities that our physical therapist recommends that you might enjoy adding to your daily routine.

- ***Walking***

Walking is one of those perfect activities that doesn't require any special equipment and is extremely practical. Why waste fuel on a short drive when you might get some fresh air and low-impact exercise instead? Walking improves the circulation without putting undue strain on your body. It also moves the weight-bearing joints, which is particularly beneficial if you have arthritis.

- ***Running***

Running is harder on the heart, lungs, and knees than walking, but these demands can be beneficial to your wellbeing. The well-known "runner's high" that you might have read so much about seems to have its own pain-relieving properties for chronic pain patients. The adage "no pain, no benefit" seems to apply here as well. Running's routine can allow your brain to lower its pain sensitivity baseline, making your other aches and pains seem less bothersome.

- ***Cycling***

Cycling would get you to your destination while still providing you with a variety of health benefits. The aerobic workout will help you improve your heart health, while simply riding the bike will improve your balance and leg strength. Cycling is also lower-impact than running if you have back pain or knee issues.

- ***Swimming***

If even walking is too much for you these days, a swim in the pool could be a better option. Since water reduces the effects of gravity on the body, swimming is extremely beneficial for people with arthritis or extremity injuries. And if you can't swim, try some water-based walking or dog-paddling.

- ***Weight training***

It's not enough for "muscle-heads" to lift weights. Weight training will assist in the growth of muscle tissue that supports your joints. Muscles that are stronger are less prone to fatigue and painful strains. Training with weights also helps you retain your bone density to prevent muscle wasting as you get older.

As part of a well-balanced physical therapy regimen

You can do any or all of these things on your own time, or ask our physical therapist about incorporating them into a full-fledged physical therapy program. If you're rehabilitating an injury, uncertain of your exercise tolerance, or dealing with a chronic pain problem, the latter approach may be particularly beneficial.

Our physical therapist will assess your health and recommend activities that are appropriate for your needs and goals. At the same time, other healthy, beneficial modalities such as massage, ultrasound therapy, dry needling, cold and heat treatments, acupuncture, or laser therapy can be able to improve the benefits of your activities. These treatments can help with tissue recovery, inflammation relief, pain relief, and the desire to keep going and have fun.

Life's too short to waste it in your bed or chair. Get up right now and make an appointment at our physical therapy facility. It's the healthiest decision you can make!

PART V

~HOW TO PROPERLY COMBINE NUTRITION WITH SPORTS FOR A HEALTHY LIFESTYLE~

The standpoint between good nutrition and good health is well-known. Food and its effect on athletic success has become a science in and of itself.

A nutritionally adequate diet is the basis for better results, whether you are a competing athlete, a weekend sports participant, or a committed daily exerciser.

Dietary criteria for regular training

The basic training diet should be adequate to meet the following requirements:

• provide sufficient energy and nutrients to meet the demands of training and exercise;

• improve adaptation and recovery between training sessions ;

• provide a wide variety of foods such as wholegrain breads and cereals, vegetables (especially leafy green varieties), fruit, lean meat, and low-fat dairy products to improve long-term nutrition habits and behaviors;

• provide enough fluids to maintain maximum hydration before, during, and after exercise ;

• support the athlete's short and long-term health.

The diet of an athlete

An athlete's diet should be close to that prescribed for the general public, with energy consumption split as follows:

- ✓ More than 55% carbohydrates;
- ✓ 12–15% protein;
- ✓ Less than 30% fat.

Individuals who exercise vigorously for over 60 to 90 minutes a day may need to raise their carbohydrate intake to 65 to 70% of their total energy.

More recent recommendations include carbohydrate and protein guidelines based on grams per kilogram (g/kg) of body weight. Many athletes should adopt fat intake guidelines similar to those provided to the general public, with a preference for fats derived from olive oils, almonds, avocado, nuts, and seeds. High-fat foods such as cookies, cakes, pastries, chips, and fried foods should be avoided by athletes.

Carbohydrates and physical activity

All carbohydrates are catabolized into sugar (glucose) during digestion, which is the body's main energy source. Glycogen is made from glucose and is processed in the liver and muscle tissue. It can then be used as a primary energy source to power exercising muscle tissue and other body systems during exercise. Athletes will improve their glycogen reserves by consuming high-carbohydrate foods on a regular basis.

If a person's carbohydrate intake is reduced, his or her ability to exercise is harmed because there isn't enough glycogen stored in the body to fuel the body. As the body can begin to break down muscle tissue to satisfy its energy needs, this could result in a loss of protein (muscle) tissue, which can increase the risk of infections and illness.

Carbohydrates are required for both energy and recovery

Carbohydrate specifications are currently recommended based on the length, frequency, and intensity of exercise. Wholegrain breads and cereals, which are high in unrefined carbohydrates, can form the base of an athlete's diet. More refined carbohydrate foods may help to increase total carbohydrate intake, particularly for people who are very active.

Athletes can change the amount of carbohydrate they eat for fueling and rehabilitation based on their level of exercise.

Consider the following scenario:

- Light intensity exercise (30 minutes a day): 3–5 g/kg/day;
- Moderate intensity exercise (60 minutes per day): 5–7 g/kg/day;
- Endurance exercise (1–3 hours per day): 6–10 g/kg/day ;
- Extreme endurance exercise (over 4 hours per day): 8–12 g/kg/day.

Glycemic index and athletic success

The glycaemic index (GI) assigns a score to foods and beverages based on how carbohydrate-dense they are and how easily they affect blood sugar levels. In the field of sports nutrition, athletes are becoming increasingly interested in the GI.

More study is needed to validate the best sports nutrition guidelines. Low GI foods, on the other hand, can be beneficial before exercise to provide a more sustained energy release.

Foods and fluids with a moderate to high GI score can be the most effective during exercise and the early stages of recovery. However, it's important to note that the type and timing of food consumed should be adjusted to the individual's tastes and to maximize the person's success in the sport in which they participate.

Meal served prior to the excercise

The athlete's pre-event meal is an important component of their pre-exercise training. Threc to four hours before exercising, a high-carbohydrate meal is thought to improve efficiency. A small snack one to two hours prior to exercise can also help you perform better. Some people can have a negative reaction to eating prior to an exercise session. A high-fat or high-protein meal is more likely to cause intestinal distress. Meals rich in carbohydrates and known not to trigger gastrointestinal distress are suggested just before exercise.

Pre-exercise meals and snacks include cereals, yoghurt, and pasta with tomato sauce. Examples of suitable pre-exerption are cereals and oatmeal, toast or muesli with a small sauce, or muesli, and fruit salad with low-fat creamed sauce.

Eating when exercising

An intake of carbohydrate is needed during exercise lasting more than 60 minutes to maintain blood glucose levels and delay exhaustion. According to current guidelines, 30-60 g of carbohydrate is appropriate, and can be consumed in the form of lollipops, sports gels, low-fat muesli, sports bars, or white-bread sandwiches.

It is essential to begin your intake early in the exercise session and to consume consistent amounts during the workout. To prevent dehydration, it's also necessary to drink plenty of water during long workouts. Water, diluted fruit juice, and sports drinks are all good options. Up to ninety grams of carbohydrate per hour is recommended for people who exercise for more than four hours.

Eating after a workout

Following exercise, it's important to replace glycogen quickly. After exercise, carbohydrate foods and fluids should be consumed, particularly in the first one to two hours. Eat carbohydrates having moderate to high GI in the first half hour or thereabout after exercise to replenish glycogen reserves. This can be done before the daily meal schedule is restored.

Sports drinks, juices, toast, low-fat milk, low-fat flavored milk, sandwiches, pasta, muffins/crumpets, fruit, and yoghurt are all good places to start when it comes to refueling.

Sporting efficiency and protein

Protein is an essential component of any training diet, since it aids in recovery and repair following exercise. Since many foods, especially cereal-based foods, are a combination of carbohydrate and protein, a high-carbohydrate diet may generally meet protein requirements.

Sporting people should consume significantly more protein than the general population.

As an illustration:

- ✓ The daily recommended amount of protein for the general public and healthy people is 0.8–1.0 g/kg of body weight;
- ➢ An individual of 60kg can consume 45–60 g protein per day;
- ➢ Non-endurance athletes should eat 1.0–1.2 g/kg of body weight each day if they exercise everyday for 45–60 minutes;
- ➢ Athletes participating in endurance and strength competitions – those who exercise for longer periods of time (more than one hour) or who engage in strength training, such as weight lifting, should eat 1.2–1.7 g/kg of protein per day.

According to dietary surveys, most athletes can easily meet, if not surpass, their protein needs by eating a high-energy diet. As a result, taking protein supplements is unlikely to help you do better in sports.

Other issues associated with very high-protein diets, though more research is needed, include:

• increased cost

- a possible negative effect on kidney function
- increased weight if protein options are also high in fat
- a lack of other healthy foods in the diet, such as bread, cereal, fruit, and vegetables.

Enhancing athletic efficiency with dietary supplements.

Your vitamin and mineral requirements are fulfilled by a well-planned diet. Supplements are only useful if your diet is lacking or if you have a diagnosed deficiency, such as an iron or calcium deficiency.

Extra vitamin doses do not increase athletic performance, according to research.

Vitamins, minerals, spices, meal supplements, sports nutrition products, and natural food supplements are all examples of dietary supplements, which can be contained in pill, tablet, capsule, powder, or liquid form.

Before you start taking supplements, think about what else you can do to increase your athletic performance – diet, training, and lifestyle improvements are all more tested and cost-effective options.

Supplementing with vitamins and minerals can be harmful as well. Supplements can only be used under the supervision of a licensed health practitioner. Instead of using a supplement or pill to fix nutritional imbalances, it is preferable to evaluate and adjust the diet.

It's also crucial to note that, no matter what level of sport you participate in, taking supplements puts you at risk of breaking anti-doping rules.

Sporting capacity and water

Dehydration can affect athletic ability and, in the worst-case scenario, lead to collapse and death. It's very important to drink lots of water prior to, during, and after exercise. Don't wait until you're thirsty to get something to drink. Fluid intake is especially necessary for activities that last longer than 60 minutes, are intense, or are held in hot weather.

While water is a good choice, sports drinks can be necessary, especially in endurance events or in hot weather. The sodium in sports drinks aids absorption. In sports nutrition, a sodium content of 30 mmol/L (millimoles per liter) seems appropriate.

It is no longer recommended that you use salt tablets to treat muscle cramps. The muscle tissue is affected by a lack of water, not sodium. Zinc or magnesium deficiency may be causing persistent muscle cramps.

What resources are available for assistance?

• The doctor; Dietitians Association of Australia, 1800 812 942; Sports Dietitians Australia, (03) 9926 1336

• Eating well will help you do better in sports.

• A well-planned, balanced diet should provide enough protein to support muscle growth and repair while still meeting the majority of an athlete's vitamin and mineral requirements.

• The diet should be based on foods that are high in unrefined carbohydrates, such as wholegrain breads and cereals.

• Athletes should drink plenty of water to improve efficiency and avoid dehydration.

PART VI

~HOW NECESSARY IS SLEEP FOR THE BODY'S RECOVERY?~

Who doesn't like a good night's sleep that is both relaxed and restful? It's good news. The doctor prescribed quality sleep, the kind that leaves you looking refreshed and feeling energized. Sleep, like food, nutrition, and exercise, is vital to your health. The right amount and quality of sleep, regardless of age, enhances focus, actions, memory, and overall mental and physical health. Many essential functions of the body are maintained and controlled by sleep, the most important of which is restorative. More than at any other time, our bodies use the time provided by sleep to repair cells and tissue, develop muscles, and synthesize proteins.

There are many health benefits to having the right amount of sleep, but there are just as many significant health risks of not getting enough.

Even a two- or three-hour reduction in the ideal eight hours per night will significantly increase the risk of developing any of the following:

- Alzheimer's disease

- Cardiovascular disease
- Immune dysfunction
- Depression
- Diabetes
- Hypertension
- Obesity
- Accident susceptibility

Sleep problems could affect your mental health by affecting your habits, body sensations, attention, feelings, and even your thoughts. Unsurprisingly, a lack of adequate sleep has been related to a reduced lifespan over time. Sleeping less than five hours a night has been shown in several studies to increase mortality risk by up to 15%.

Despite this, many of us underestimate the possible implications as our lives become increasingly crammed with familial, educational, and other events, cramming more and more into our days and nights and leaving quality rest as an afterthought.

Sleep deprivation is a rising problem that affects people of all ages. The correlation between a lack of sleep and car and industrial accidents, as well as medical and other occupational errors, is becoming stronger.

Your lifestyle and career may also have an effect on the quality of your sleep. Adjusting to a normal sleeping pattern after a sleepless night or trip-induced jet lag can normally be accomplished with some deliberate planning; however, for physicians, nurses, pilots, construction staff, and other shift workers, or others who deal with major schedule disruptions on a daily basis, it can be considerably more difficult for their natural internal clocks to stay healthy. Working shifts that alternate between days and nights can throw off the cues that your body uses to control when and how long you need to sleep, such as light or a lack thereof.

Life decisions may also have an impact on how well you sleep. Any parent will attest to the huge effect that a new baby or teething toddler can have on keeping a regular sleep schedule (or even having any sleep at all!). Extracurricular and family events become increasingly evening affairs as children reach kindergarten. According to the National Sleep Foundation, "scheduled evening activities [are] the most popular obstacle to getting a good night's sleep" for both children and adults, with 41% of parents and 34% of kids having trouble getting a good night's sleep at least once a week.

Sharing sleeping quarters or living with someone else may have a significant effect on sleep. It's not unusual for the other partner's sleep to be disrupted or disrupted while one partner is having trouble sleeping. According to a new North American poll, 76% of those married or living with someone said their partner had at least one episode of insomnia in the previous year, with 33% claiming their partner's sleeping issues are causing problems in their relationship.

SIGNS THAT YOU ARE NOT SLEEPING WELL

How do you know if you're not getting enough sleep?Or, even more importantly, if you're getting the kind of sleep you need to be your most creative, happy, and balanced self?

Aside from just feeling tired, there are a number of indicators that you aren't sleeping as well as you should be.

The following are a few of the most common:

Excessive daytime sleepiness, exhaustion, or lack of energy, which may lead to the need to nap or disrupt everyday activities.

Feeling exhausted or unrested when you wake up.

It takes longer than 30 minutes to fall asleep or you have trouble falling asleep in general.

Frequently waking during the night or difficulty sleeping.

Not being able to get back to sleep after waking up too early.

Sleeping too much or too long can mean that the quality of your sleep isn't up to par.

HOW TO GET BETTER SLEEP

While your life may appear to be constantly busy, and your current sleeping habits, arrangements, and consistency are less than optimal, there is still hope! There are many ways to enhance your sleep, and actively implementing even a handful of them would almost certainly result in a more restful and pleasant night's sleep.

Make a calming evening routine

Establish a pre-sleep routine that relieves some of your everyday stress by doing things that calm you. A routine may eventually serve as a signal to your brain that it's time to sleep. When you wind down, try meditating, breathing exercises, or listening to relaxing music, or try other calming practices like meditating, breathing exercises, or listening to soothing music. Maintain a routine that requires a consistent sleeping schedule.

Even on weekends, keep your meals, bedtime, and morning alarm consistent. Maintaining your sleep schedule trains your body to anticipate and react to acceptable periods of rest and wakefulness.

Make your bed a relaxing haven

It makes a difference what you sleep on. According to research, a new bed will increase a night's sleep by up to 42 minutes and is more successful than sleeping pills. This is possibly due to the structure of a bed over ten years old degrading by up to 75%, causing sleep disturbance and potential spinal pain. As you begin your path to better sleep, consider purchasing a new mattress or bed. Experiment with numerous pillows to find the one that is perfect for you. Make sure your mattress is on a slatted foundation for greater air circulation and less sweating.

Sleep in your room and sleep alone

Electronics, food, and other relaxing activities should not be allowed in your room. This will cause the brain to brace itself for sleep rather than eating, reading, watching TV, playing video games, learning, or talking on the phone when you lie down.

Take all electronics out of your home. Electronics and screens have become an inseparable part of our everyday lives. Televisions, computers, tablets, phones, and other interactive devices are significant sleep disruptors due to the behaviors associated with them, the light they produce, and the stimulation they offer. Keep gadgets out of the bedroom and unplug at least an hour before bedtime.

Maintain a peaceful, calm, and dark environment in your bedroom. To mimic your ideal sleeping conditions, remove light, sound, and maintain a constant temperature in your room. Consider installing noise-canceling carpeting, installing light-blocking blinds, or wearing an eye mask to reduce visual disturbances if necessary. Caffeine and alcohol should be avoided.

Caffeine can be avoided in the hours leading up to bedtime, but even during the day. While some people may get away with a morning cup of coffee, others can note that the effects of caffeine last long into the evening. Remember that caffeine isn't just in coffee and tea: it's also in soft drinks, cookies, over-the-counter drugs, and herbal remedies. To ensure that you're mindful of your regular caffeine consumption, read the labels or chat with your pharmacist. Alcohol is considered to affect overall sleep quality and worsen respiratory difficulties as well as restless arms and legs.

Exercising is necessary

Exercise is a well-known stress reliever, and people who exercise regularly (30-60 minutes, three days weekly) sleep better and are happier overall. Obesity, a significant risk factor for sleep deprivation, sleep apnea, insomnia, and daytime sleepiness3, is also combated by exercise. Exercise, of course, is a natural energy booster, so get your workout in at least a few hours before bedtime. Avoid taking naps. Although a fast "power nap" can work wonders for some, it's safer to stay awake during the day if you're having trouble sleeping. This helps your body and brain to predict and adapt to a daily waking and sleeping schedule. If you really must sleep, limit it to 30 minutes or less.

On a full – or empty – stomach, stop going to bed. Balanced, nutritious meals during the day will help you sleep better by keeping your body and blood sugars in check. Make an effort to stick to a meal schedule and avoid eating big meals right before bedtime. If you are hungry, eat a light but healthy snack (low-fat dairy or turkey) that won't fill you up and will give you a boost of energy. To boost the odds of having a good night's sleep, avoid high-fat foods like popcorn, ice cream, and fried foods.

If you cannot sleep after 30 minutes, get up. After a half-hour, you really can't sleep? Don't be concerned. Be kind to and generous with yourself. By waking up and resetting stuff, you can relieve stress and anxiety. Before going back to bed and then trying again, leave your room for a while and return to some of your pre-bedtime relaxing practices or routines. Make it a top priority, and then schedule it in. According to a recent North American poll, it takes an average of 23 minutes to fall asleep; if you're concerned about your own sleep, you'll probably need as much time, if not more, to fall asleep. As a result, keep in mind when making plans. Committing to getting the sleep you need (and using the methods to get it) can necessitate some significant changes in how you eat, function, and even play, which can be difficult at first. Do not give up! Note, those extra few hours will support the mind and body in a number of ways.

The importance of sleep cannot be overstated.

CONCLUSION

It's not easy to lose weight or live a healthier lifestyle in general. Most of the time, we make the decision to live a healthier lifestyle, but we can't help but slip up now and then. DETERMINATION is the secret to leading a happy, balanced lifestyle, and as simple as the word sounds, it entails a lot.

You must be able to ignore unhealthy things, no matter how appealing they can seem, because most of the time, we simply pile on the calories and don't get to expend even a quarter of them.

You must be determined to live a thin, happy, and free life. Yeah, indeed! You're unstoppable, so go for it.

Do Not Go Yet; One Last Thing To Do

If you enjoyed this book or found it useful, I'd be very grateful if you'd post a short review on Amazon. Your support really does make a difference, and I read all the reviews personally so I can get your feedback and make this book even better.

Thanks again for your support!